Midlife Mamas On the Moon

Celebrate great health, friendships, sex, and money and launch your second life!

Sunny Hersh

Celebrate life! Sunny

Fast Forward Publications
Long Valley, New Jersey

This book is intended as an entertaining introduction to topics in health, relationships, life decisions, and finances in midlife. It is not intended as a substitute for medical evaluation or treatment by your doctor, and is not a substitute for competent professional financial or psychological advice. The author and publisher do not recommend starting any new treatment, changing any medication you may be taking, or using over-the-counter preparations without consulting your personal physician. This book is intended for educational purposes only, and use of the information is entirely at the reader's discretion. The author and publisher cannot be responsible for any adverse reactions arising directly or indirectly from the suggestions in this material, and disclaim any liability from the use of this book.

Published by
Fast Forward Publications LLC
Post Office Box 573
Long Valley, NJ 07853

©2004 by Sunny Hersh

Cover design by Jenn Theiller
Book design by D.J. Todd
Photography by Lorenzo Gasperini
Cataloging-in-Publication Data
Hersh, Sunny
Midlife Mamas on the Moon: Celebrate great health,
friendships, sex, and money and launch your second life!
International Standard Book Number 0-9743093-7-0
Library of Congress Card Number 2003108940
1.Middle aged women—Health and hygiene
2. Menopause
3.Hormones
4. Middle age—humor

Printed in the United States of America   1 2 3 4 5 6 7 8 9 0

Dedication

This book is dedicated with love and thanks

To my fantastic husband, Scott
and my children, Aviva and Asa,
my three best friends in this world,

To our loving Creator,
our best friend for all time,

And to my Mom and all the
women I know or will know.

Thank you for your courage,
friendship, and persistence—
you inspire me every day!

Introduction

We're not over the hill— we've moved the hill back!

That bulge in the population that was born between 1946 and 1964—the baby boomers—has decided that the 40's and 50's aren't old. For the Midlife Mamas of today, 40 is the new 30, and in your 50's, you're just getting started! Instead of rocking on the porch, we're rocking the world with our entrepreneurial spirit, savvy work style, independent approach to aging and health, and enlightened focus on relationships. Throughout most of human history, most women died by the age of 40, so it's obvious that we're blazing a trail through uncharted territory. In the 20th century, our great-grandmothers, grandmothers, and mothers have been the guinea pigs for the new longer lifespan, showing us how to—and how *not* to—navigate through the additional forty-some years we've been given.

Imagine your 40's as the infancy of your second life.

Life changes quickly in the years between 40 and 60, yet this is when we build the foundation for later years. Midlife Mamas have so many choices, so much pressure, and so many demands competing for their time and energy that we sometimes feel paralyzed by the need to sort out the information flying in our faces at warp speed. How do you lose weight, reduce stress, eat the right foods, lower your blood pressure, raise great kids, have great sex, balance your hormones, advance your career, and prepare for your financial future while keeping all your everyday balls in the air? How can you *create* a healthy, happy future rather than *reacting* to random events?

Let me be your guide to the wonderful doctors,
natural healers, financial planners, psychologists,
web sites and wise writers
of all types who have focused their amazing spirits
and expertise on the rest of your life!

Let's build joy, bust stress, boost hope, and come up with some quick fixes and long-term solutions. Let this book be the "digest," the beginning of your exploration of the many choices that are open to you. Use "The Checklist" and "The Check-up From the Neck Up" at the end of each chapter to jump off into new areas of interest. Say "The Checkup from the Neck Up" to yourself to make your resolutions real. Photocopy the lists and put them on your refrigerator, on your computer monitor, and in your purse as you go to the market, the doctor's office, the library, the bookstore, and the Internet. Love yourself enough to create the fantastic future you deserve.

See that your joys and concerns are shared
by so many other Midlife Mamas.
We've all made it to the moon,
but we're just beginning to reach for the stars!

VI.

**Is she positive because she has a great life,
Or does she have a great life
because she's positive?**

Dear Midlife Mamas,

*Yes, my friend Sunny Hersh has a great life, with an outstanding circle
of friends, a prosperous business, two gorgeous kids, a powerful husband
who loves her, and a great story to tell you about yourself in this book. But
not everything about Sunny's life has been sunny.*

*Her happy childhood ended suddenly when her father's business went
bankrupt, her father had a paralyzing stroke on the day of her high school
graduation, and her mother had a nervous breakdown shortly after. She
and her brother were faced with decisions no teenagers should have to
make. She made a decision at that time to focus on the bright side of things
and to develop habits that would support that view—no matter what.*

*Her first year of college had already been paid for, so she went, studied
hard, met Scott, and struggled to return, despite her parent's decision that
she should abandon her dream of graduating from college. Opportunity,
preparedness, and blessings united, and she got a full scholarship to return,
work at every part-time job she could find, graduate, and marry Scott.
Just when married life was getting predictable, they had their daughter
Aviva and started a business that took off like a rocket.*

Sunny has always had a smile and a good word for everyone she meets, and supports my efforts to empower women to be successful in their lives and their businesses. When she speaks to groups, she shows people how to have a good time while learning something. My husband and I guided them, but they were the kind of associates who always did more than they needed to do and were ready in 15 minutes to go wherever they needed to go.

When Sunny lost her vision and her mobility in a head-on collision, she wouldn't allow anyone to even speak of the possibility that her health wouldn't return. It did return, and she and I became pregnant at the same time, but then she had a series of miscarriages related to the accident. With characteristic determination, she pressed forward with unpleasant fertility procedures and gave birth to her son, Asa. During all these struggles, she steadily built her business and dealt with the long illness and death of her father. Then her mother succumbed to depression and was in and out of psychiatric hospitals and nursing homes until her death.

Through it all, Sunny never misses an opportunity to laugh, celebrate something with her children, or give someone a compliment. **I told you about her struggles so you know she has created a great life because she interprets events in a positive way.** I hope you'll pretend you're having coffee and talking with her while you read this book and kick off the second half of your terrific life.

Claudia Nardone, CFO, Nardone Associates, Inc.

VIII.

Read Midlife Mamas on the Moon a la carte, in any order you like. Just read whatever grabs you today.

Introduction IV
We're not over the hill—we've moved the hill back!

1. **Reinterpret Your Life Story—**. 1
Use it to Ignite Your Next Life

2. **Garbage in-Garbage Out** 9
Don't let your mind *talk* to you like that!

3. **Lose Weight with your Eyeballs** 20
Bracelets, books, and the old listeroo—
the secret is really between your ears!

4. **The Absolutely Free, Totally Guaranteed,
Fat-Burning, Ab-Toning Fountain of Youth Pill – Vitamin X!**. . . . 35
(If only you could put Xercise in a pill.)

5. **Is Your Life Worth 30 Minutes a Day?** 49
Answer yes and get consistent.

6. **Devour and Conquer—**. 57
Anti-aging Food Factoids You Can Use

7. **If you ate like a monkey, you wouldn't
need supplements, but do you?** 66
Supplements, water, and sleep to take life to the next level.

8. **That was very 9/10 of you!**. 78
Stay on the high road with a continuous positive
program of vision and laughter.

9. **Raising Kids—** 87
Not a true - false or a multiple-choice test, but a never-ending essay

10. **Empty Nesters and Boomerang Kids** 95
Just when you get used to the empty nest, they're baaa-aaack!

11. **Last Chance Midlife Mommies** 106
Hey-I'm 40 and I forgot to have kids!

12. **Husbands and Wives, Best Friends to the End** 109

13. **Losing Your Virginity—** 124
The second time around

14. **Sexual Fitness** 134
Use it or lose it.

15. **What Goes Around Comes Around—** 145
It may be your turn to be Mom & Dad to Mom & Dad

16. **Friends Help You Love Your Life—** 152
Be the best friend you'd like to have.

17. **Soaring Solo** 161
Living large, with a side of guys!

18. **Anything worth doing is worth doing now!**................. 169
Change careers, sail around the world, open an inn, become a minister?

19. **It's My Perimenopause, And I'll Cry If I Want To!** 180

20. **Get It While You're Hot!** 191
There is an alternative to the dangerous HRT you've heard about.

21. **Natural Hormones** 201
Stop Denying and Start Flying

22. **Go With the Flow**.................................... 209
Keep that urinary tract flowing and glowing

23. **Will Power and Your Financial Diet** 215

24. **Let Your Ripples Loose!** 231
Serving the world, and the kid next door

25. **News Flash—90% of Heart Disease Is Due to Lifestyle Choices** 236

26. **What's up Doc?**...................................... 248
Do you plan your healthcare as carefully as your next vacation?

27. **Boning Up For Your Future** 258
Osteoporosis—Be afraid, be very afraid

28. **Your Laugh Lines Prove You've Had More Fun Than Your Kids.** . . . 263
Is Mom visiting you every day—in your mirror?

29. **Loss—Getting Beyond "Why Me?"**...................... 275

30. **Start From the End & Look Back**....................... 281
When you have to decide what's important, it's usually
what you already have.

31. **Have a Thick Skin and a Thin Heart** 288
Forgiveness lets you live more fully.

32. **Keeping the Faith** 293
BIBLE—Basic Instructions Before Leaving Earth

33. **"To Pray is to Work, To Work is to Pray"** 303
Believing that prayer heals the mind and the body is easy

1.

Reinterpret Your Life Story— Use it to Ignite Your Next Life

"Will your personal life story in Second Adulthood be conceived as a progress story or a decline story? To a large degree, you have the power of the mind to make that choice. Yes, you will encounter losses in Second Adulthood, some of them irrevocable. But you will also have the accrued experience and judgment to adapt to them along with the confidence of a firmer identity and far greater self-knowledge than you ever had in First Adulthood. You also have a greater capacity to love and to be loved, in ways far deeper and less selfish than when you were younger. The opportunity is to get on with the real work of your Second Adulthood—the feeding and crafting of the soul."
New Passages: Mapping Your Life Across Time, **Gail Sheehy**

On Sunday afternoon, February 9, 1964, I set my hair with Dippity-Do and huge juice cans and put a blue net over it. I was getting ready for the really big show – the Beatles were going to appear on "The Ed Sullivan Show" at 8 pm. I wanted to look good for Paul (the cute one), George (the shy one), and John (the smart one), even though I'd just be watching in my girlfriend Nancy Hartwell's living room. During the show, we screamed, ate cheese doodles, and made her dog Fritz bark. What was my dream back then? Was it to actually "be with" one of those guys (did I know what that meant?), or to just be in the crowd watching them, screaming, with my hair looking large?

Remember the big dreams you had at 8, 18, and 28? At 8, you dreamed you'd grow up to look like Barbie. At 18, you knew you'd become an actress, famous architect, or amazing entrepreneur. At 28, you imagined a fantastic, exciting life with this guy you'd married. At 48, you're hoping to get more fiber in your diet and stay awake long enough to watch Letterman. Your kids may be the same age as The Beatles when they appeared on Ed Sullivan, and the AARP will soon know your name. What happened? How did your mind go from confident dreaming to barely living day to day? How did fear win out over the love of a great life?

Is it fear or is it love?

When you think about it, one or the other motivates everything people do. When you wonder why people do things, take it down to love or fear. Your son burns you a CD of your favorite music? He loves you. Your mother-in-law never recognizes your holiday preparations? She fears *her* daughter won't measure up. Your old friend doesn't call and stay in touch? He fears you will judge him because his business failed. This kind of thinking cuts through layers of anger right through to your compassion—*they* may not even realize it's fear, but now that *you* do it's easier to forgive and move on. Your husband empties the dishwasher and vacuums the kitchen? Either he loves you, he's a double and aliens abducted your real husband, or he wants to have sex. Simple, huh?

Your memories of fearful events and failures can't be erased, but you can have power over them. Often fear stands for **F**alse-**E**vidence-**A**ppearing-**R**eal. Think of the factors that make you more or less fearful. Why do you drive instead of flying? Terrorism

is a new, out-of-control threat, but statistically driving is a much bigger risk. Why do you eat the cheeseburger, knowing that heart disease is more likely to kill you than West Nile Virus, breast cancer, or a nuclear accident? Why are you more afraid when someone else is driving drunk, than when *you* are? The actual risk is the same or greater, but you feel safer when you're in control.
So much that we fear is in how we perceive it.

If God's going to grant your wildest dreams, you've got to *have* some wild dreams!

When you were a little girl, fear kept you safe from busy streets, hot stoves, and biting dogs. But as an adult, fear can keep you in your comfort zone, guarding you from potential rejection and disappointment and telling you to stay in boring jobs and bad relationships because they're "safe." Fear doesn't know you want meaningful work and relationships. Fear tells you not to face bad thoughts, and to numb them with food, alcohol, drugs, cigarettes, and overspending. Fear tells you not to take a risk until you have the degree, the perfect mate, the promotion, the kids are older, the skinny body – all the things that we mistakenly think will guarantee that if we *do* take a risk, only good things will happen. **Fear keeps you doing the same things over and over again and expecting different results—and that's the definition of insanity!**

The truth is that in order to move from fear to freedom, we have to take carefully considered risks. Once you realize the events from the past that are crippling you, you can start the small acts of courage that will move you forward. Even a turtle makes progress only when he sticks his neck out! Don't let old fears govern your life. Reinterpret the events in your past—bad and good—as stepping-stones to your current awareness. When you reinterpret your life, you'll be able to decide what your mind loves to think about, what you value about yourself, and let your actions move toward that.

I'm a much better dreamer now than I was back in *Meet the Beatles* days. Now, my dreams are stoked by people I love passionately, with details I've learned by living life—not by images on a screen. Your dreams are the same—the passion and colors that flesh out your dreams today make them vibrate. They attract the information and support you need from all sources, heavenly and otherwise. (That's called "grace.") See a pattern now in the formless "wants" you used to have; it's as repetitive and vivid as a symphony or a movie you've seen and loved. Choose to love the form that your life has taken, rather than dwell on what it could've, would've, or should've been.

Watch out for fear junkies. These are the people who know everything wrong with everything and why everything won't work. They don't mean to do it. They are toxic and you can't save them. If they're an unavoidable part of your life, try to recognize when they're talking from fear and don't take it personally. Remember, layered under negativity, hatred, and aggression, you'll find fear. Know who you *can* go to for advice in important areas of your life, and make good use of their time by doing your research, making lists, and taking notes.

What's on your "Life is Short, Start Now" list?

Right off the top of your head, you can probably come up with three or four things you've always wanted to do and a couple of places you've always wanted to visit. You may want to finally learn to swim, ride a horse, play the guitar, or take a cooking class. Leave a yellow legal pad laying around over the weekend and expand that list into 100's of things! Don't put any limits on your list based on how much time you have or what you can afford. Start four files:

- A **Dream** File, with pictures of **things** you'd like to own, inspiring words, and articles from magazines

- A **Life is Short** file, with pics and info about **experiences** you
  will have, like taking a balloon ride over the Napa Valley
  or building low income housing in Guatemala
- A **NOW Project** file, with details, Internet searches,
  photocopies from books on **three things you're
  working on now**
- And an **Other Projects** file, with random clippings
  on ideas for the future.

At first, the files will just hang there in their little crate with
nothing in them. But you'll be surprised how quickly they'll fill
up with glossies of tropical vacations, articles from the Sunday
paper, and lists of places you can go hiking with your family.
This book started with an empty file named Book.

Know and conquer your "distractive habits."

Excessive TV-watching, e-mail checking, talking on the
phone—they're not destructive to any one but you and your
dreams. But they are "distractive" because they distract you
from what you really want to do. Compulsive eating, sleeping,
and shopping are ways to numb your awareness and hide from
your true destiny. They keep you from spending that time alone
with yourself, with a pen and pad, discovering the steps that will
lead you to where you want to go. All you have to do is be
aware that you're doing it again—catch yourself in the act—and
consciously put down the catalog you're dawdling over, get off
the internet and get on with productive things. Real relaxation
is good, but these "distractive" habits are just mind-numbing junk.

Kids believe in the Tooth Fairy, Dora the Explorer, a choo-choo
train made out of boxes, and wishes that come true if you blow out
all the candles. You can be a believer, too. Don't let your mean
boss, your ex-husband, or even your beloved sister who went and
died on you take that away. (Your sister would want you to have lots

of fun and excitement, so go ahead and have a dream in her honor!)

How can I be such a Pollyanna when there's a hole in the atmosphere and children starving all over the world? I can interpret my life and the life of this world as a project that's moving forward because it's the right thing to do. All the great writers say so, including the awesome writer who said, "A woman without vision shall perish!" Not "a woman without money," not "a woman without good health," not "a woman without a good education"—it's the woman without a positive vision who will be blown away by life's accidents! If your vision is right, it will always be bigger than the junk that comes along and the mistakes that you make. When you reach your wit's end, but you have a big dream for the future, you'll…turn right!

If you're raising a child with health, learning, or developmental problems, you must always hold a vision of that child as an independent, happy adult. Develop a vision of what you'd like your marriage to be like. Flesh out the dream of your own business and keep your senses open for clues of how to make it happen. Pursue your art with passion and others will want to see it. Know that even though you've made mistakes, you're worthy of your vision. And when you know exactly what you want, the circumstances will surface if you're ready to recognize them.

Every setback is a setup for a comeback.

Even 9/11 can add a positive direction to your life; here are some of the good things that came out of 9/11 for me. I notice beautiful natural things and my blessings more often, and thank God frequently for them. I always say, "I love you" now when I say goodbye to a loved one, knowing that goodbye *could* be for real. I don't put off loving gestures. I stay in touch with the people I love and plan to spend good times with them, and I make those plans *before* I get my work done. (My work gets done anyway.) If I think of something

I meant to say, I say it or I call right back and say it, even if it makes me look foolish. Hurt feelings, compliments, hard questions —I put them right out there, so there's no unfinished business. I've always loved my country passionately, but now I plan to put my hands to work in solid projects, along with my heart.

The Checklist

❏ **I.** For more about the simple universe of love versus fear, read *Love is Letting Go of Fear*, a wonderful little book by Gerald G. Jampolsky, M.D. Instead of harboring anger and fear and waiting for your enemies to attack, you see the advantages of a full frontal attack of loving unconditionally.

❏ **2.** Wander around on Oprah's website, oprah.com— she is an expert on taking the best message out of your own life, and teaching others to do the same. Register for the "Live Your Best Life" interactive workshop, the online version of Oprah's Spring 2003 five-city tour. Learn how to run your brain for the better! Don't whine because you don't get home in time for her show; record it or watch rebroadcasts on Oxygen.

❏ **3.** Leave that pad out on the counter and start writing your "Life is Short, Start Now" list today. Don't be afraid! What's the worst that could happen? You won't get what you wrote down? It's fun just thinking about it, and your mind will begin to guide your life to what you want. Someone laughs at you? Great—now you know who's holding you back.

❏ **4.** Using the results of your "Life is Short, Start Now" list, write a fifty-or-less word statement of your objective as if it's already true. Here's mine: My family is healthy and wealthy in love, moving forward in life with joy in all things! I am a successful author, helping thousands of women love themselves enough to take positive action!

The Checkup from the Neck Up

❑ I am a woman of vision, taking steps toward my dreams each and every day. It's me against me, and the best part of me is winning!

❑ When I look at my life, I see a tremendous work in progress, with each good and bad event along the way invested with meaning and purpose.

❑ I've learned that taking risks is part of the game, failure is never final, and freedom is never free.

❑ Living life to its fullest is a decision, and I've made it!

2.

Garbage In—Garbage Out Don't Let Your Mind *Talk* To You Like That!

"What you have now is more freedom – an additional choice. You can choose to use optimism when you judge that less depression, or more achievement, or better health is the issue. But you can also choose not to use it, when you judge that clear sight or owning up is called for. Learning optimism does not erode your sense of values or your judgement. Rather it frees you to use a tool to better achieve the goals you set. It allows you to use to better effect the wisdom you have won by a lifetime of trials."
<u>Learned Optimism, How to Change Your Mind and Your Life,</u>
Martin E.P.Seligman, Ph.D.

Would you agree that you're influenced by the people you hang around with? Any parent or anyone who's ever worked in an office would have to agree with that. But what if I told you that **the person you talk with the most is you?**

Seventy percent of the conversations you have each day are with you. Your thoughts are the conversations you're having with yourself and your feelings about your life come from the way *you explain your choices to yourself.* But you don't *have* to obey every thought that comes into your head; you can and must control your self-talk. One of the oldest authorities on effective living, the Bible, tells us the importance of this in the phrase "As a woman thinketh, so shall she be."

When you control your words, you control your thoughts.
When you control your thoughts, you control your soul.

Are you focusing on what you *can't afford* or what you *will have*? Are you saying you're enjoying terrific health or declaring you "don't want to be sick?" Are you imagining yourself in your new home or screaming "I can't live in this place anymore!" Are your conversations filled with proof of how badly your industry is in the dumps or peppered with examples of new opportunities you've found? Are you a victim of fate, luck, karma, the economy, the government, your parents, your boss, or God? Or are you put on this earth to fully experience joy, freedom, and prosperity? You deserve *all* those things, and I believe you're born into this world with the intention to feel good and attract good things. Don't let negative words and stinking thinking derail you from your destiny; your intention to be happy and hungry for life is not selfish, it's true to God's design.

Cut the Stinking Thinking!

Thoughts are also beliefs, beliefs that may have come from an overcritical father, a jealous sister, or a burned-out teacher. You were young, you were vulnerable, and you accepted these statements as facts. If you've said "I'm just not organized/creative/athletic/a good student" or any other of those self-judgments, do you think you were born that way? Or was it *said about you* at some point, and you believed it? Ask yourself "Is this perception really a fact, or was it something I picked up somewhere?" Remember that every crime against humanity began as a thought!

Most of today's parents know they shouldn't compare their children, but how many times have you heard someone say, "She's my shy one/smarty-pants/tomboy"? When I was 13, 5'8" tall and 135 pounds, my mom would agree with people when they pronounced me "a big girl." I still wince when I hear that label. (And of course now I'm thrilled to stay around 135 pounds.) My son Asa's dyslexic struggles with reading and writing have been mediated by years of special education and he jokes about the "sped" label, but Scott and I and his label-defying teachers have drilled him with the self-worth message for so long that he's pulling 4.0's at college. So many of the things we think about ourselves are things others have said about us, not facts.

In *Learned Optimism*, Dr. Seligman writes about the things pessimists think when they explain negative events to themselves:

- The pessimist's problem is permanent (diets never work),
- it's pervasive (I'm disgusting), and
- it's personal (I'm just a weak person).

The optimist tells herself that *her* problem:

- is temporary (life is stressful right now),
- specific (ice cream is my favorite),
- and external (being at a party makes me eat more).

The double whammy Dr. Seligman sees is when the pessimistic style combines with "rumination"—obsessively analyzing problems, failures, and defeats over and over again, like a cow chewing it's cud. It's a combination of blaming yourself for outcomes and believing that outcomes will usually be negative. These behaviors get passed down in families and can end in full-blown depression. By age 11, it's already more common in girls than boys.

Argue With Yourself

How can you change your pessimistic thoughts and your tendency to constantly focus on problems? In Seligman's model of "flexible optimism," you learn to argue with yourself. When you eat the Extreme Ultimate Blizzard Sundae when out with friends, you don't say to yourself "I dieted for two weeks, and now I blew it! I might as well eat everything in sight, because my friends must think I'm a fat slob and they're totally right!" Instead, the Midlife Mama says "Whoa, that was not a good choice! I didn't eat dinner, so my total calories aren't that much higher. I ate well for two weeks, and I can go back to doing that. My friends ate junk food too, so we'll all laugh about it. It doesn't make sense to eat more junk, so I'm just going to go right back to my healthy eating. I'm concerned about my bad choice in that situation, but I'll work on it." You've turned yourself around without putting yourself down.

If you're one of those obsessive thinkers whose negative thoughts go round and round like clothes in a dryer, **try a physical or imaging technique to shift your attention.**

- Snap your fingers or snap a rubber band worn on your wrist.
- Pretend your mind's a TV, and switch the channel to happy thoughts.
- See yourself as a Queen, controlling the kingdom of your mind.
- Imagine painting a big red X across the intruding face or image.
- Write your concerns and blessings down on two sides of the same page.
- Sweep the negative thoughts away with a SWISH of your hand.
- Think of your brain as a jukebox, and press the button to play joyful songs.

Banging on a wall, carrying a red STOP sign in your pocket, or focusing on a peaceful beach or holiday scene are all attention-shifting strategies to stop your mind from clinging to pessimistic thoughts when they serve no purpose (which they usually don't).

The goal is to learn to pull away from problems temporarily, strategize some solutions, and put them into action without over thinking.

Do you feel lucky?

I hope so, because people who *think* they have good karma usually *do* get luckier than the rest of us. They sincerely believe love and money are coming their way, and they say things like "I always win at card games." Because these lucky ducks are more optimistic about their chances, they follow their hunches, take more risks, and keep trying. When something good comes knocking on their noggin, they think they deserve it, so they tend to follow up and act on the opportunity. If the optimist's sweetheart hit the road, someone new is right around the corner! Laid off from the job? Karma chameleons let go—and move on to a new career.

It's thimble time!

It's helpful to have some handy phrases to say to yourself and others at life's challenging moments, and you can use the ones in the chapter-endings, The Checkup from the Neck Up. Howard Kaminsky and Alexandra Penney have collected some fun and well-honed phrases in *Magic Words: 101 Ways to Talk Your Way Through Life's Challenges*. My favorite is "It's thimble time," what you say to yourself when someone says or does that really annoying thing—*again!* Let's say you have a physically fit friend who continues to make little comments about your weight and erratic exercise routine ("It's a shame I have to run that 10K without you") even though you've brought your irritation to her attention. You tell yourself that **it's thimble time**, time to protect your attitude from those meaningless little jabs that could ruin a great friendship, just as a thimble protects your finger against needle pricks. How about "**Let's quit while we're behind**" if you see that a discussion is going nowhere? Flummox the familiar time-is-money phrase that urges you to rush ahead; say "**Time is honey**," instead, reminding yourself to appreciate the everyday blessings and savor the precious commodity of time spent doing meaningful things.

Your refrigerator can be Positive Image Central.

I plaster mine with happy family photos, pictures of dream vacations, meaningful poems and prayers, funny greeting cards, and lists of important goals, foods, and supplements. Houseware stores sell plastic frames with magnets to keep everything clean. Children's art is another favorite display. A positive refrigerator is like a giant billboard in the center of your home, broadcasting what's right about your life and your goals for the future. My children were horrified recently when the refrigerator was stripped for cleaning. "Are you okay, Mom?" they asked, concerned that all was not right with the world when the refrigerator had no happy pictures.

"But all this positive thinking stuff is just crap!" you say. "It's just not reality and it's not the way I was brought up." Hey, if your family members model the exact life that you want to live, go ahead and duplicate everything they do and say. It's not a matter of denying reality, it's a matter of **what you *choose to focus* on**. It's a reality that 3,000 people died horrible deaths on September 11th because of some religious fanatics. But do you focus on photos of people jumping from the building, or stories about heroes and families going on with their lives and honoring their loved ones? Choosing what to focus on is something you're already doing; refining the process of making choices is a skill you can work on.

Think of your brain as a computer.

Programmers have a saying about input and results—garbage in equals garbage out. If you watch a lot of negative television, constantly listen to angry talk radio, read trashy violent novels, and never miss the sensationalized evening news, you probably won't be a calm, spiritual person who thinks outside the box. How could you be? You're putting garbage in your mind, and garbage will come out of your mouth and show in your actions. When I go to a comedy club, I find myself thinking of curse words for days afterward. Young people whose friends have many sexual partners and watch shows where the characters are promiscuous begin to accept the behavior as "normal." Researchers find that children who watch more violence on television are more aggressive.

My 23-year-old daughter pointed out recently that we had stopped taking our own positive-speaking advice! Running down a list of recent financial reverses in the sluggish economy, Scott and I thought we were explaining why we couldn't provide an exciting family cruise vacation. What she perceived was a woe-is-me attitude. Her prescription was for us to once again count our many blessings and enjoy the view while riding the Staten Island ferry together—for free!

In a Yale School of Medicine study, researchers studied the impact of people's opinions on their health. They found that the most accurate predictor of these 2,800 people's survival over the next ten years was the answer to the question "What do you think about your health?" In results that controlled for preexisting conditions and behaviors like smoking, **people who said their health was poor were seven times more likely to die than those who said their health was excellent!** In another study, lab rats implanted with tumor cells died or got sicker if they had been conditioned to believe they were helpless.

The Spoken Program—Erase It by Replacing It!

One of our family's favorite fairy tales is the story of The Two Sisters at the Well, derived from the bible story of Rebekah at the well. The kind sister draws water for the wizard disguised as a helpless old lady, while the mean sister refuses to help her. The wizard causes flowers and precious jewels to flow out of the mouth of the kind sister, and frogs and snakes to leap out of the mouth of the mean sister each time she speaks. It's powerful to imagine the words coming out of your mouth as diamonds or toads, making the world sparkle or shrivel!

Your words and thoughts are the most potent programmer of your own brain. When one of our family members predicts a bad outcome (It probably won't work, I'm not good at that), we tell each other "Don't speak what you don't want!" *Never* predict negative outcomes in your future like "My daughter has such a strong personality, she'll be out of control as a teenager", or "My husband is so focused on work, he'll never learn to relax."

Neuroscientists using brain scans have identified increased connectivity in brains when positive words were heard, and noted that thoughts or words that are repeated create new pathways in the brain. Seniors who repeat positive words about aging such as "wise" and "experienced" can walk faster and are more coordinated. A 1999 study found that changing behaviors is best done by focusing on the benefits of the new behavior, not the negative consequences of the old.

The shortcut to loving yourself and taking positive action

**is to write down specifically what you really want *as if it has
already happened,* and read it, listen to it, visualize it, or say
it out loud repeatedly over time.**

I'm not saying you should lie to yourself about some unreachable
ambition. Saying "I am the Queen of England," or "Ben Affleck
can't wait to meet me" will *not* produce those desired results! It
must also be specific and personal to you; the old "every day in
every way, I'm getting better and better" doesn't work as well as
the kind of affirmations you can personalize from this book.
Self-talk expert Dr. Shad Helmstetter explains that the

"...use of self-talk should not be confused with earlier
concepts of simply maintaining a 'positive attitude.' The use of
Self-Talk is, instead, the application of specific self-directives
which are worded in a specific way in order to achieve a
predetermined result through the natural processing and
response functions of the human brain."

Helmstetter, the author of **What to Say When You Talk to
Yourself**, goes on to counter the idea that self-talk is
"brainwashing," which uses rewards and harsh punishments to
control thoughts and behavior. Today's self-talk is personally
directed by you, to get you out from under the thumb of a
lifetime of negative external programming. You don't even
have to believe in self-talk for it to work; if you continue to
shake up your pathways with the positive new words and
thoughts, it will help in spite of your skepticism.

Prayer may be the ultimate affirmation!

Telling your brain what you want it to think is a form of prayer.
You are substituting thoughts of faith, truth, beauty, and success for
the old nasty ones of fear, anger, worry, confusion and depression.
Look through the prayer book that you read as a child, and see
words that say you will "go out in joy and be led forth in peace,"

or that your "strength is made perfect in weakness." Yes, you may find some of the images of an angry or restrictive God that scared you when you were little. Are you seeing them through the eyes of some past authority figure, or through the eyes of the smart, strong adult you've become? Search your heritage, a new faith you're attracted to, or write your own prayers, acknowledging that a higher power can be your partner in throwing your whole self into your over-40 brain control project!

The Checklist

❑ **I.** Pick up the TV schedule and decide what you want to put in your precious brain. Is it a contest, documentary, or drama that shows the best of people or their very worst side? Do you feel uplifted after you watch it? New fascinations I've noted are public embarrassment and humiliation masquerading as "reality," and the graphic depiction of dead bodies, usually those who've died violent deaths. Is that a productive focus for you and your family? Be careful about cop/lawyer shows; they often show good guys dealing with filth, but you're still exposed to the filth. Do you really want to know details about serial killers and pedophiles?

❑ **2.** Songs have a powerful self talk effect for two reasons: they often repeat a phrase over and over ("I believe I can fly"), and setting words to music has a powerful memory effect. You prove that's true when you remember a song from second grade but can't remember why you walked down to the basement. Make up a special CD for yourself on *itunes.com*, stock up on spiritual music, or order the *Instant Party* or *Pure Disco* CDs.

❑ **3.** Positive books are mentioned throughout *Midlife Mamas*—put the ones that appeal to you on the "wish list" you can make on Amazon.com. For a fresh monthly jolt of positive, I like *O: The Oprah Magazine, Prevention,* and good old *Reader's Digest* (great source of clean jokes.) *Woman's Day, More,* and all the women's magazines are very life-affirming, which says a lot about women, doesn't it? *Men's Health* is great for the man on your list, and *USA Today* is the most upbeat newspaper.

❑ **4.** There are thousands of books about the continuous loop between your mind, your mouth, and God, but here are the classics: any and all versions of the bible; *Man's Search for Meaning,* Victor Frankl; *Think and Grow Rich,* Napolean Hill; *Tuesdays with Morrie,* Mitch Albom; *The Power of Positive Thinking, You Can If You Think You Can,* Dr. Norman Vincent Peale; *Move Ahead with Possibility Thinking,* Robert Schuller

The Checkup from the Neck Up

❑ As a woman speaks, so shall she be!

❑ I create my awesome life with my positive words, thoughts, and actions.

❑ My words affirm everything that is great about me, my family, and the universe!

❑ I think and speak the best as if it has already happened, creating a positive loop between my mouth, my mind, and God!

3.

Lose Weight With Your Eyeballs

Bracelets, Penny Pinching, the Divided Dish, Books, Magazines, and the Old Listeroo— The Secret is Really Between Your Ears!

"If you wear a size zero, do you exist? Are dressing rooms fitted with fun house mirrors? Does the acid in diet soda destroy the calories in pizza?...If men had menopause, would there be a 'little blue pill' for hot flashes that was fully covered by health insurance?"
—<u>Today I am a Ma'am</u>**, Valerie Harper**

"Never eat more than you can lift."—**Miss Piggy**

"I never got my figure back after giving birth, and that was fifteen years ago. I didn't really want my figure back anyway, I wanted someone else's."—**Anonymous**

"Eat all you want, just don't swallow it."—**Joan Rivers**

Have you ever heard of the 80/20 rule? It's in the Murphy's Law showcase of truisms. You wear 20% of your clothes and shoes 80% of the time. A mere 20% of your work output creates 80% of your income. 20% of the people in any organization do 80% of the work and make 80% of the donations. **The work of weight loss is also in an 80/20 configuration—80% is calorie restriction and 20% is exercise and energy output.**

This was bad news to me after I hit 40 and gained 20 pounds. I'd already established a fun exercise habit, and those who've met me know I love to put my energy out there in every direction. I've tried to bargain with the 80%; **maybe if I just eat lots of healthy foods I can eat as much as I want.** I felt virtuous spreading hummus on my bagel instead of cream cheese, and sopping up olive oil instead of butter on my Italian bread. Olive oil has no cholesterol, but it's 120 calories a tablespoon. Hummus has no saturated fat, but almost the same number of calories as cream cheese. Whole grain bread has more fiber than white bread, but sometimes has *more* calories. "Eating healthy" is important and encourages mindfulness, but it's not the whole answer to weight loss. An extra 100 calories a day of input and 100 calories less of output, and you're 10 pounds heavier in one year.

The other common bargaining ploy is to believe **you can "exercise it off," eat as much as you want, and not gain weight.** 18-year-olds and winners of the Naturally Lean Gene Pool Lottery have a maddening ability to do this, but not most women over 40. Writing down, balancing, and limiting the amount of what you eat is the inescapable answer to 80% of the weight loss equation.

By the time you reach 40, you've probably tried several of the latest fad diets—been there, done that, bought the T-shirt, donated the book to the library. The diet might have even been a fun experience, something you were excited about and shared with co-workers or friends, competing with each other to lose the most weight. Then, real life crept in and you gained the weight back, usually with a few extra pounds. In your thirties, you could starve yourself or work off the weight, but now those short-term strategies don't seem to work as well. The real answer is painfully obvious – permanent lifestyle change. You're very aware of what you need to do, which is to eat less, choose healthy foods, and exercise. Ugh. Someday, a substance like gut hormone PYY will help us curb our appetites and be slim like everybody on Star Trek and the soap operas, but for now we're left with personal choice.

What you *used* to do to *lose* weight may now be what you need to do to *maintain* your current weight. You'll only find that out if you begin, persist, and succeed with a healthy program. **If 65% of American adults are overweight or obese, the problem is not that you are a weak-willed, ineffective person.** Our entire culture is struggling with processed foods served up in huge portions to people who now spend many hours of every day in front of a TV, a computer screen, or a car windshield. Is it the inactivity, the 800-calorie Frappuccinos or the 700-calorie tuna sandwiches? In the 70's, 1 out of 7 Americans was overweight; in the 90's, 1 out of 4; today, it's 2 out of 3. The guy who invented super-sizing discovered three things: people will pay more for a larger portion and eat up to 30% more; but they feel like pigs going for a second portion. You may laugh (I know I do) when people sue McDonald's or the makers of Oreo cookies for making them fat, but it indicates how desperate and powerless people feel. Maybe we *do* need the Fat Police to storm the house when we eat Double Stuff Oreos and milk, but it doesn't seem cost effective, does it?

Limiting or temporarily cutting out alcohol is a major secret to successful weight loss. Your alcoholic beverages have almost as many calories as pure fat — but they're worse!

Instead of signaling your body that you're full, alcohol calories say "Hey, let's have some fun, some chicken wings, and some taco chips!" They slow down your metabolism for days and a hangover cuts down on your enthusiasm for your exercise program. Wine is better than sugary margaritas and rum in diet cola beats martinis. Try this – cut your intake in half, drink a glass of water for each glass of whatever, and resolve to be the life of the party anyway!

Forget the concept of "blowing it"—you'll just use that as an excuse to eat junk for three days. When you fall off your horse, named New Lifestyle, just get right back on and keep riding into the sunset. Try asking the **HALT** questions: Am I **H**ungry? Or am I **A**ngry, **L**onely, or **T**ired? Beating yourself up about eating something "bad" is responsible for more extra pounds than fast food! Then there's the mindset of "Let me just have some of this-and-this-and-this before I go back on my diet!" (That can last a week.) Water is New Lifestyle's favorite beverage, since fruit juice, sugared tea, and non-diet soda have too many calories and don't fill you up like solid food. I drink some diet soda, but what *is* it, really – a chemical cocktail?

Break up 3 meals into 5 and have The Second Lunch.

Stop saving all your calories for dinner and skipping breakfast and lunch! That slows down your metabolism because your body thinks it's starving. If you can do it, eating only three times a day is great. **If you *start* eating only three times, you only have to *stop* eating three times,** and stopping is usually the problem. Having meals at 8 a.m., 2 p.m., and 8 p.m. works, but doesn't fit into normal schedules. My husband can do this but most women need to eat every four hours, **saving something from each of those three meals for the late afternoon and the evening, keeping blood sugar levels on more of an even keel.**

Have an open-faced sandwich at lunch and have the other slice of whole wheat bread with some peanut butter and sugar free jelly at 3 p.m. Think of it as four, five, or six 300-calorie meals. (Somehow, the name *snack* brings out the empty carbs.)

Save your after-dinner fruit for 8 p.m. Eat it in the kitchen, and make a new rule that no food is allowed in the TV room – you will break the association between TV watching and snacking. Nonfat light yogurt (Dannon Light n' Fit – 90 cals.) is a great, calcium-and-probiotic- rich, easy snack. Trans-free popcorn, walnuts, and almonds satisfy, but only if you can stop at a few and not gobble down the whole package. I can't stop shaving little slices of cake, and Scott can't stop spooning light ice cream or frozen yogurt, so *we* can't keep those in the house; you may be different. The idea is to write down what you eat and **break up those *same* calories throughout the day.**

It helps to think of that late afternoon snack as The Second Lunch. That means it is about 100 to 150 calories and has some protein, like yogurt, string cheese, cottage cheese, egg whites, a veggie patty, peanut butter, or half of a protein bar, to chase those grumblies away until your vegetable-rich, sit-down dinner. Changing how you eat is a **step-by-step change in how you *think* about eating** – as fuel for your awesome Maserati-racehorse-world-blessing body.

Get some sleep! You know exhaustion makes you a sissy when facing those 4 p.m. cravings, but it also makes it harder to keep your fat-burning furnace stoked. Weight-related hormones like glucose, cortisol, and thyroid go haywire when you're sleep-deprived.

Bracelet Bingo – Strive for Five, but Nine is Divine!

Mindfulness is another important key to weight loss, since so much of our eating behavior is automatic. A crucially important first step is absolutely knowing how many fruits and vegetables you are getting in a day.

Yeah, yeah, I eat my veggies, you say. But do you really? **A fun mindfulness strategy that helps you lose weight with your eyeballs is wearing rubber bands or bracelets, and switching them to the other arm after each plant-based food is eaten.** If your initial goal is 3 veggies and 2 fruit, you switch the 5 bracelets on your left wrist to your right wrist as the foods are eaten. I picked up 3 sets of 3 elastic bead bracelets in blue and silver at Wal-Mart. (I'm such a matchy-poo fiend that I had to wear blue for three days until I got over myself.) Flesh colored rubber bands would be less conspicuous, but less mindful as well. My friend Sara lost 6 pounds in the first 2 weeks of bracelet-switching, and needless to say had no constipation problems on 9-a-day!

Or instead of a penny for your thoughts, how about a penny for your pounds? Nine pennies can be moved from one side of the counter or one pocket to the other, or you can use quarters and buy a new pair of shoes when you've eaten 9/day for 30 days. Your eventual goal is 5 veggies and 4 fruits. (As *Prevention* magazine experts say, "strive for five, but nine is divine"). Getting that produce in doesn't happen by accident—if you fail to plan, you're planning to fail. Stock up on ready-to-eat veggies and keep fruits out where you see them as reminders.

The Divided Dish and other Diet Deception Detectors

Grab a paper plate and a marker or crayon. Draw a line across the center. Then divide one of the halves in half. If you're eating to lose weight, model your plate of food after the divided one by filling up half your plate with veggies or salad and the small sections with a serving of lean protein and one of whole-grain carbs. Having that plate around reminds you that

1) a big mound of spaghetti with a jot of broccoli on the side is not dinner and 2) the meat serving should be smaller than the veggie serving. Little paper plates and bowls keep servings small and the sink empty. Don't feel full? Wait a few minutes to let your brain register the food, and you can always have a salad with a spritz of olive oil and vinegar or a sprinkle of original Newman's.

Sugarless gum is a great tool for those who eat while they're cooking, driving, or watching a ball game or a movie. You have to consciously sabotage yourself, take the gum out of your mouth, put it in a napkin, and grab the food (and then it tastes weird). There are those who chew gum and eat, but let's not go there. It's not classy to chew gum at a party (Didn't I meet you at the bowling alley?), but try holding a wine glass with ice, club soda, and a lemon at all times. You'll attract others who know the Extreme Water lifestyle (you'll all have lots of chats on the way to the bathroom).

Keeping a food diary – that's an actual list of what you eat —is a powerful weight loss aid. You can keep it simple by writing what you ate on a legal pad, and add it up at the end of the day. You can use one of the logs in the Cruz, Karas, or Greene books, or you can use *The Pocket Food and Exercise Diary*, available on Amazon. You may have tried and failed with the old listeroo in the past, but try again, because this simple tool really works.

With visual reminders, you *see* very plainly that you've reached your goal, and you snap that last one over with the same satisfaction you feel when the taxes are done, the project is finished, or that last dish is in the dishwasher and the counters are clean! My daughter used "manipulatives" like this in her student teaching, since students learn better when touch and feel are combined with seeing and hearing. So will you!

Other helpful visuals:

Serving of meat, fish or chicken	=	deck of cards or cassette tape
Cup of cooked rice or pasta	=	tennis ball
Serving of cheese	=	four dice
Serving of peanut butter	=	ping pong ball

The eyes of coworkers are upon you for many, if not most, of your waking hours. Why not use *those* eyeballs to lose *your* weight? Your Benefits Manager may be the first one to talk to about a group weight loss program, because she may know of free incentives offered by your health care provider. Coffee breaks and lunches are built-in support meetings, and it's easy to share tips and organize a 20-minute walk. Group momentum and competition come into play with a weight-loss contest – start with a weigh-in of participating members of, for example, the sales versus the public relations department, with a prize at the end of six weeks for the *highest overall percentage* of weight loss. Talk about downsizing! Sweets will disappear from the office, and birthdays will be celebrated with a tray of strawberries.

"Take off 20 Pounds of Ugly Fat in Two Weeks!"

Got your attention, didn't I? And so does every magazine out there, screaming at you to walk off weight and fight fat with this tip and that food, promising the final solution to that nagging weight problem. Are they telling the truth? Are they doing you a favor?

For the most part, yes. When they offer suggestions from successful weight losers, trainers, health spas, diet books, research findings, diet doctors, and celebrities who take advantage of all of the above—they are usually offering you valid strategies and inspiration to move forward on that goal, though they tend to emphasize quick-sounding solutions. They are desperately sifting through complex studies and product/ press release materials to find the stuff that actually may work for you. They know that good information will keep you listening to their message – and to their advertisers.

Besides, what's the worst that could happen? If you go on the *Woman's World* Soup Diet this month and the *First for Woman* Okinawan Formula next month, you'll eat more veggies and fish and lose weight – is this bad? Think of it as cross training for dieters!

Almost half the people surveyed by the American Dietetic Association, the largest organization of dietitians in the US, said they get their nutrition information from television and magazines. That's why the American Council on Science and Health, a watchdog group of independent scientists, had nutrition experts examine the 20 highest circulation magazines for wild claims, accuracy, and sound science. As reported in *The Better Life Institute Letter* online, "The most significant finding was that none of the magazines received a "Poor" rating, the first time that's happened. The authors attribute that to an emphasis on the science behind the nutrition instead of just headline-grabbing fads. The general interest magazines that were judged to be "Excellent" were *Parents, Cooking Light,* and *Good Housekeeping.*"

Bestseller Diet Books—They all work!

Like you, I've done them all, from Atkins to Pritikin to South Beach. I've gorged on bacon and steak (my big toes hurt —I got gout) and I've stayed up until 2 am making healthy soup without a speck of fat for the next diet day. I've enjoyed hanging out with Suzanne Somers in my kitchen and getting to know her family. And I've lost weight on all of them, **because they all force you to focus on what you're eating instead of shoving random food into your mouth! They often involve** shopping and cooking, which promotes loss because restaurant meals are usually 30% larger and fattier than those you cook at home. They keep you focused on their particular "secret" while you cut back on eating junk with no food value. The postscript to the story is, of course, that if old habits resume, diets don't work. **Changing your eating and exercise habits from now until forever is the real deal, and you and I both know that we've got to increase our emotional fitness in order to do it and keep doing it.**

Do **Atkins, South Beach, and Somersizing** work? Yes, because they use the principles that protein and fat help you feel full and empty-carb white pasta, bread, potatoes, soda, and sweets that spike your insulin must be curbed. It's all about the greens, grains, and protein—the South Beach Diet (healthy people's Atkins) has you cutting the whole grains, fruit, and dairy for two weeks and then gradually bringing them back in with your lean protein, good fats, and veggies. They all recommend that you cut out caffeine and alcohol for a period of time, and that alone will make a huge difference for some! I didn't feel well on Atkins, but I found Somersizing effective. Suzanne's recipes are delicious, she loves to *eat,* she's an advocate of bioidentical hormone replacement, and she has integrated her love of food, cooking, and sharing meals with friends and family into her lifestyle. Her son-in-law is her personal trainer and friend, and her husband loves to eat the way she eats. What could be better?

At first glance, Jorge Cruise's *Eight Minutes in the Morning* seems like an "exercise book," as you will find two exercises per day for 28 days pictured in it. Morning strength training is the core of the program, but every aspect of weight loss is covered in the most concise, positive style in this excellent program. Cruise uses all the state-of-the-art motivational techniques to fire up an excellent eating/exercise regimen—a before & after picture & body measurements, Success Chart, a Success

Contract you sign to yourself and people who'll support you, daily pep/info tips and Eating Cards that detail your intake.

Seems like a big rigmarole, but if you've tried and failed and think constantly about losing weight, I guess you *need* a big rigmarole, right? His eating program incorporates the top current thinking, including:

- out with saturated and trans fats, in with omega fats, flax oil, and olive oil
- in with lean protein from fish, chicken, egg whites, & soy
- out with the white stuff, in with whole grain breads, cereals, and brown rice
- unlimited vegetables and a piece of fruit
- cut the sugar, caffeine, and alcohol

Veteran personal trainer of Diane Sawyer and other notables, Jim Karas hammers away at the most important tool you've got for weight loss and maintenance—your attitude. In *Flip the Switch*, he outlines all the excuses you've ever used— your schedule, your gender, your genes, your job—and shows you how to overcome them and finally face reality and take responsibility for your actions. It's like having a kind, funny trainer who hears what you say (and this guy has heard it all) but gently points you on the right path with an eating and exercise plan and a shopping list. He's got you watching portion sizes while eating in the real world and keeping a food diary. He doesn't want to hear about your thyroid, your bad genes, or your big bones. Get a blood test, determine how to deal with your family profile, and take off the pounds so you can actually see if those bones are big or not. It's calories in versus calories out. Period.

The other guy in the Super Trainer Triad is Bob Greene. Oprah's trainer and author of *Get With the Program and Make the Connection*, Bob is the Accountability Guy, helping you chart your progress through emotional eating and ever-increasing movement. His spiral-bound book is very easy to use and packed with thoughts on why we eat what we eat and what to do about it.

Another great book to help you on this journey is Dr's Michael Roizen and John La Puma's *The Real Age Diet: Make Yourself Younger With What You Eat*. This is an awesome mindset that you can use every day of your life. **When you eat something, does it age you or make you younger?** Imagine picking up a cheeseburger and thinking, "This is making me older." The whole trend that you see in the media today about power foods and living younger because of food choices comes from Dr. Roizen's first *RealAge* book, now rounded out with 80 delicious recipes in *Cooking the RealAge Way*.

Good old **Weight Watchers** has been around for ages because it works! Applebee's restaurants teamed up with Weight Watchers to create a lean menu for those who want to skip the mucho nachos. Kind of retro, "something your Mom did," but it uses the power of group psychology to show you how to watch your weight, discussing why you succeeded or failed with like-minded folks each week. Cuts the crap and the excuses when you have to weigh in and say it out loud, know what I'm saying? **Studies show that the group support, flexible points program, and leaders who've been successful with the diet are a combo that helps people lose three times the weight and keep it off.** The points program allows you to eat or drink at a party, for example, but you plan for it earlier in the day by sticking to zero point vegetables and salad. Go on weightwatchers.com and enter your zip code to find the nearest meeting you can sample; though they offer an online program, I'd go with the human contact version. Unlike some other plans, you can pay as you go and there are no contracts. *Weight Watchers Make It in Minutes* cookbook has 200 quick recipes on the plan.

Meal Substitutes? Yes, they can work because you don't

handle food, and portion sizes are controlled. There's a service that uses this principal now by shipping perfectly prepared Zone meals and snacks to your home for about 40 bucks a day—and they wonder why weight is becoming a class issue! I'd stay away from the high-carb supermarket brands of bars and shakes and go for higher protein versions. Most find that high protein substitutes like Revival Soy and Nutrilite Protein Bars work best, with protein grams above 15. Labeling laws changed in 2001, forcing high-protein foods to include body-unavailable glycerin carbs. Some companies cheat and some include them, so check to see that *available* carbs are below 15. When you just don't have access to a yogurt, salad, or turkey-on-wheat sandwich, shakes and bars are better than a cheeseburger or greasy Chinese food from the food court.

The Checklist

❑ **I. Prevention magazine is at the center of the healthy universe** with invaluable advice in every area of health, weight loss, nutrition and more. Just subscribe to it, for real or online, and don't give me any lip that your mother gets it—she's no dummy. The *Nutrition Action Healthletter* is another great one. My favorite feature is the Right Stuff versus Food Porn on the back cover. Entries from the *Nutrition Action Newsletter's* "Right Stuff"—Blue Diamond Almond Toppers, Del Monte Packaged Greens, Mann's Sugar Snap Peas, Burger King Veggie Burger, Wendy's Salads.

❑ **2.. Sugar substitutes** have never actually been proven to help people lose weight. But if you like to use them, Sweet n' lo and Splenda (sucralose) appear to have fewer side effects, though the saccharin in Sweet n' lo has been known in studies to hang around in animal organs. In the health food store, ask for stevia, an herbal sweetener from South America. I got joint pain, my friend Audrey got migraines, and many other people complain of reactions to Equal (aspartame), though tests show it to be safe. Suzanne Somer's Somersweet is a pared-down, delicious form of fructose. If you're pregnant, I'd stick with sugar.

❑ **3. Eating disorders** used to be a teenage affliction, but now anorexia, bingeing, purging, and laxative abuse **are on the rise among midlife women**. Women dealing with family and hormone changes feel that they can control their eating, even though everything else in life may be spiraling out of control. They say things to themselves like "I'll see how long I can go without eating" and "The thinner I am, the younger I look." Obsessive exercising also helps the sufferer hide from other emotional issues. Women who've been treated as teenagers are at especially high risk. Antidepressive drugs like Celexa have been shown to help binge eaters. Residential treatment with long-term follow-up is recommended. If you or someone you know needs to understand the seriousness of this mind set and its treatments, read the heart-wrenching book *Slim to None,* by Jennifer Hendricks.

❑ **4. Antidepressant drugs and progesterone often increase appetite;** as your mood rises, so does your appetite. Fight back with exercise and healthy eating.

❑ **5. Most weight loss supplements are useless, and ephedrine can kill you, so stay away.** A moderate amount of caffeine, as in coffee or sugar-free energy drinks like Quixtar's XS, can suppress appetite. Carb blockers and chromium picolinate may normalize blood sugar, and there is evidence that both chromium and CLA, an essential fatty acid, favor lean muscle development. Spend your first diet dollar on high quality food, your second on some strength training items, and your third on high quality supplements.

❏ **6.** Best quick ways to **dress up steamed or microwaved veggies**, 1/2 of your New Lifestyle plate—I Can't Believe It's Not Butter spray, Mrs. Dash seasonings, onion and garlic powder, or a spritz of a good oil like Enova, olive, or flax using a Misto sprayer. Sauté with garlic and onions—fresh is great but pre-minced is good too. Toss cut up peppers, asparagus, onion slices, zucchini, whatever, in a little olive oil, sprinkle with garlic powder, and broil on a foil tray or foil-covered cookie sheet in your oven to make roasted veggies. Cook in low salt broths or orange juice instead of water. Look for low-fat-*and*-sugar salad dressings.

❏ **7.** Mix things up—kick off your campaign with two weeks of two meal substitutes/day, move to a week of salads and veggie soups, alternate days of 12-15-&1,800 calories—**diet schizophrenia can be your friend**, as long as calories in are less than calories out. The low-carb lifestyle has variety now too, with products like Joe Bread (2.5 carbs) and other substitutes at low-carb stores online and the freezer in your health food store.

The Checkup from the Neck Up

❏ I've got this weight thing down—now I click past the Food Network to the Style Network! I like looking this way more than I like high-calorie foods.

❏ I leave food on my plate, now, just like the skinny people—I leave bites for the angels!

❏ I don't bring foods I can't handle into the house "for the family" any more. My family is too good for that junque!

❏ I am impressed with the new, smaller me but others may not be. We're all impressed with the loving, generous, fantastic life I'm creating.

4.

The Absolutely Free, Totally Guaranteed, Fat-Burning, Ab-Toning Fountain of Youth Pill— Vitamin X!

(If only you could put Xercise in a pill)

"Weight training strengthens your body and allows it to function at a higher level by making you capable of doing more work. I don't just mean allowing you to lift more weight; strength training will increase your ability to perform your aerobic exercise at higher levels as well, which will further decrease your percentage of body fat. You'll also get the aesthetic benefit of toned muscles. But one of the most important yet often overlooked benefits of strength training is in the way it combats two of the most profound effects of the aging process: the loss of muscle and the loss of bone mass (osteoporosis). Strength training is the best way to fight both."

<u>Get With The Program,</u> **Bob Greene**

Why does it seem harder to lose weight with each year over 40? Because it is! Simply stated, if you don't use your muscles, you lose a pound of muscle mass every year, which decreases your metabolic rate, which translates into 2 lb of fat every year. It's a simple but deadly process. That's why the exercise prescription for those over 40 has changed from "Go for a walk" to "Throw in a bit of cardio with your strength training"—about 30% cardio and 70% strength training.

You've finally found the shortcut—strength training! (There's also a shortcut to the shortcut). If you're a complete beginner, you may need to start with some stretching and walking just to begin feeling like a person with a body. The positive feelings of being outdoors and breathing deeply will help you get ready to incorporate this vital activity into your program. Jorge Cruise's book *8 Minutes in the Morning*, great for beginners, starts your weight training immediately—four sets of two exercises every day. You'll see improvement if you train twice a week, but **three times a week is the magic minimum number,** the least you can do to see rapid gains in strength and endurance. (P.S. You won't get bulky, you'll just get trimmer.)

What can a trainer do for you? Keeping you injury-free, cross-trained, and results-oriented is what a trainer does best. They're like your mother—they notice all your mistakes and they'll be quick to point out when and how you're slacking off. Charging from $25 to $75 an hour, a trainer will work with you for three weeks, three months, or the rest of your life. The expense has a "I won't eat this because I don't want to waste my money" effect, as well. I'm a little skeptical when someone says, "I can't afford something like that," and I notice their luxury car lease and expensive watch; I have to assume they're just more interested in a sleek car and a slim watch than a sleek, slim body. The trainer who works with the football team is probably not the one for you. Get a referral at a health club, from a woman your age who's found someone great, interview trainers in the yellow pages, or put your zip code in the locator on ideafit.com.

Yoga, Tai Chi, Pilates and other Meditative Exercises Are Not For Sissies and Seniors!

I know what you're thinking—weird music and lots of breathing! You're thinking there's a big learning curve, and you don't see any benefits or sweat until you practice. I thought the same thing, and I was wrong. My muscles were stretched and shaking and I was sweating within the first fifteen minutes of an Ashtanga boot-camp style class! I passed on a repetition and the class fanatic said, "You'll find it hurts more if you don't do it." Wrong—I did it and it hurt more. After class, I crawled home and assumed the corpse pose for the rest of the day. You don't have to do this stuff perfectly to benefit from it. That yoga mat can be a flying carpet to fitness. (You were right about the weird music and Darth Vader breathing, though.)

The Pilates people are really into perfection and doing things right—picky, picky, picky! That's why women who pursue it have the most amazing stretched and strong bodies, particularly those who use The Reformer, a torture rack-type machine that both supports and challenges your body. Other classes now incorporate Pilates' emphasis on The Core Muscles—abs, glutes, lower back, and hips. My biggest problem is trying not to laugh at how funny my legs and tummy look when they're shaking like jelly from the exertion! If you're a methodical, perfectionist-type person,

Pilates (privately, in class, or on a video) is for you.
BodyTrends' Pilates MatWork video is clear enough for
beginners, but kicks your butt.

You may have heard the reports that stress increases belly
fat. Chronic stress, depression, and excess alcohol
consumption cause your body to secrete the stress hormone
cortisol, which increases the belly fat related to diabetes and
heart disease. Yoga, Tai Chi, and meditation may be the key
to the flat tummy you've been wanting.

Breathing from your belly is a source of energy and spiritual
awareness in many cultures. The Hebrew *neshamah*, the Chinese
chi, the Latin *spiritus*, and the Indian *prana* all connect
breathing and spiritual exploration. Christians back in the
bible days used to hold their breath during baptism to achieve a
blissful state. *Combining* breathing, balance, and focus makes us
more graceful, and moves us toward a state of grace and inner
strength.

Considering our Baby Boomer preference for multi-tasking,
**these disciplines are the ultimate in time management—
improving fitness and opening the door to a higher power at
the same time!** In America, traditional Christians and Jews
may shy away from them, thinking their association with other
cultures might contradict traditional doctrines. **But leaders of
all faiths are finding that whatever you focus on during
meditative breathing is enhanced,** whether it's the mysteries of
the Jewish Shema, the teachings of Christ, or the peace of
Buddha.

OK—You've decided to sign up for the gym!

Whether it's a class at the Y or a big gym with lots of
equipment, the most important thing is that **you have to feel
comfortable there and want to go!** Your neighbor may have

raved about it, but when you go there, you may hate it! She may be inspired by the superfit model types in chic exercise togs, while the atmosphere makes you want to gag.

Visit at the time of day that you're committing to, whether after work, or first thing in the morning. If there are three hostile people waiting impatiently at each machine you want to try, look elsewhere. Comfortable babysitting arrangements, fun classes that stretch and strengthen in new ways, and a friend you look forward to exercising with are huge benefits that keep you coming back, the way you've promised yourself. Ask about some personal training to get you started—many clubs include it. **Don't sign anything on your first visit**; go home and think about it or visit a second time.

I always feel more comfortable in a new place if I'm dressed like the natives. Note what everyone is wearing when you visit; there's wide variation in fitness gear. At some clubs, everyone is wearing the very latest exercise ensembles, and you can pick up a reasonable facsimile at Marshall's or Wal-Mart so you'll fit in. Real fitness clothes, and especially real exercise bras, help you feel free to bend, stretch and jump. For great fitness clothes over size 14, go to Junonia's web site or call 800-586-6642. One expensive club I sampled was heavy on the corporate golf shirts and T-shirts earned at company marathons. Another club's members sported jewelry, tattoos, and logos from deli's, landscaping companies, and excavating firms. When I wore a unitard to a class at the local Y, the women wearing their kids' cast-off Long Valley Soccer League t-shirts thought I was trying way too hard.

Serious, padded sneakers replaced twice a year are a must—none of those wishy-washy old tennis shoes, please! No one cares if they make your feet look small. Used-up shoes with no shock-absorbing material can turn fitness fun into a death march. There is a comfy shoe for every size, width, and arch height. (Check reviews in *Shape*, *Consumer Reports*, and *Runner's World*.) When funds were very limited at our house, my birthday and Mother's Day gifts were always good (from a discount store or sale) sneakers. If I see a great deal, I grab them and put them in the closet for when the current shoes wear out.

Yes, some people will know a lot more about this than you do, but don't be intimidated – they had to start at the beginning too! We feel particularly clumsy in the weight room, where everyone else seems to know how to use and adjust the equipment. Enlist the help of a knowledgeable friend if there's no trainer. March or step side-to-side if you get lost in a class; modify and catch up when you can, if there's too much jumping or twisting. **There was a learning curve with your first job, your first baby, your computer—and now you'll learn to maximize your fitness time. The first month will be your "klutz period,"** but compassionate people will remember their awkwardness and help you. You must pay your klutz dues. Yes, there will be thin, chiseled goddesses who make you want to quit before you start – every club or class has them. (That proves that it works, right?) I always make a point to talk to them, because I find that very attractive women are shunned by regular women, and Barbie is always looking for a new friend.

Even if you've been exercising for years, it's important to fool your muscles and try new things. Okay, so you've mastered step class. Your body is already wise to that regimen, and isn't trying too hard anymore. Try every new Pilates/bosu ball/toning/salsa dancing/spinning/stripper aerobics/African dance class out there—you never know when you'll find a new passion! If there had been a hidden camera the first time I took kickboxing class, there would've been a special edition of *America's Funniest Home Videos*. If you are behind that mirror

I'm punching at today, you know I *still* punch like a girl, but I feel incredibly empowered by throwing those punches. I can hit, I can protect my face. Most importantly, I can bob and weave and stay standing, in kickboxing and in life.

Strategies to transform beer bellies into six packs:
- Get the form right first, then add more weight.
- Start with 8 repetitions of each move and **work your way up to 12 reps** (don't go above 8 if you feel dizzy or have uncontrolled high blood pressure).
- One set (group of reps) gains strength, **work up to three sets** to increase fat burning.
- Alternate muscle groups; for example, chest and back one day, legs the next. Abs can be worked every day, but vary the routine. Plan a bodywork routine on Health.com or MyExercisePlan.com. Buy some videos on eBay, tape TV workouts, or borrow some from the library.
- Start with a 30 second interval between sets and **work your way down to a 15 second interval.**
- Drink water, water all the time.
- Think about the muscle as you're working it—the picture on the machine often shows it. Have a picture of the muscles of the body on the wall in your home gym. We're not sure why, but **being mindful of the muscle as you work it increases your return.**
- Trainers tell you to lift for two seconds and lower for four. That's good, but **here's the shortcut to the shortcut— force yourself to lift the heaviest weight you can for 6...long...seconds and lower for 6...long...seconds!** If you can stand it, you'll see a 50% greater benefit! It's just physics—there's no swinging and using momentum instead of muscle when you do the slow lift, pull, or push.

Good music will keep you interested while you count: one, one thousand, two, two thousand. The *Strong Bear FitPrime* video combines step with heavy weights and slow movements.

- 5 pound dumbbells too little, 8 pounds too much? Use 5 for the first set, 8 for the second, and eventually you'll move up.
- Slight soreness a day or two later is normal and good. Taking your multivitamin daily and ibuprofen (if your tummy can handle it) before a workout helps avoid soreness; compression, ice, and acupuncture help soothe after.   Some aching and creakiness is caused by declining estrogen, some by osteoarthritis, but exercise helps.
- Put up a sign—**Exhale on the Effort**. Imagine the healing oxygen pumping up the muscle you're pushing or pulling with.
- Keep a very slight bend—don't rigidly lock—the knees or the elbows straight. Go for the heaviest weight you can maintain with the fullest extension; **the last two reps should be tough**.
- For ab crunches, **focus your eyes on the ceiling**, lift the shoulder blades from the floor *without* pulling on the neck or tucking the chin, press the lower back into the floor, and **pause at the top**.
- In a long program, start with the biggest muscles—the back and the legs—and end with the smaller muscles in the arms.
- A good warm up equals fewer injuries.
- **Best use of your time if you only have 20 minutes**: Warm up (walk or dance) for five, do 12 minutes of strength training and abs, three different stretches, and you're done.

Stop Doggin' It—Boost walking benefits with your brain by improving form and intensity.

Doing *anything* is better than doing nothing perfectly, but if you're walking program is blah, you can boost the benefits easily. If your eyes glaze over when trainers talk form – pay attention. You're putting the time in, so you might as well maximize it.

To improve form:
- Keep your chest lifted and chin parallel to the ground as if you were balancing a **bowl of water on your head**; then you can't jut your neck forward from your spine. I also like the image of holding a **pencil between your shoulder blades**.
- Pull **shoulders back and down**, relaxing them. No shrugging toward your ears except when you're warming up.
- Water, water all the time.
- Don't stretch cold muscles; move briskly for about 5 minutes, then stretch lower back, arms & torso, calves & shins.
- Think about **pulling your navel toward your spine**, holding in your stomach, and moving each hip forward, not rotating your torso with the stride. This is kind of a tricky triad to master, but it supports your whole body, works the abs, and takes the pressure off the lower back. Try scooting along the living room rug, legs straight in front, on your butt: you'll see how the arms, hips, and stomach can do the work.
- **Pump your arms from the shoulder**, elbow at a 90-degree angle close to the body, forward and back as if in a groove or pulling back the air, not swinging across your body. Hands should be loose and empty.

- Don't walk with hand weights; you could hurt your shoulders. I got painful "tennis elbow" using the PowerBelt.
- Have someone observe your walking; you may not be aware of bad habits.

Stop slogging along and punching your exercise time clock. Get out of your comfort zone and you'll see results.

To increase intensity:
- **Put your feet down faster**—don't take longer strides. Heel to toe, with toes pointing forward, feel your butt and thigh muscles as you push off from behind. Take heel-toe shorter steps downhill and lean forward slightly uphill.
- **Add some short bursts of jogging**—Think "I'll jog to the fourth mail box" or "I'll jog for 100 steps." Start on a trail or around a grassy playground instead of pavement, and stretch to avoid shin splints and sore hips. Go above 4.2 mph on your treadmill and up that incline in short bursts or let the program do it for you— challenge yourself and stop leaning on the handles.
- **Walk uphill, to motivational fast music, with a fast friend or a dog** that's trotting. Count and increase daily steps with a pedometer to a goal of 4,000 steps a day (about 2 miles). An ambitious goal would be 10,000 steps (4 miles) per day. A pedometer that measures steps is cool, 'cause it shows how **exercise is like coins in your pocket—it all adds up!** The $22 FreeStyle Pacer Pro (800-949-1563) or *Prevention's* Digital Step Pedometer are good ones. Some consecutive days boost overall benefits.
- **Do something different**, like cycling, a different machine or video, or a live class. Take three different classes per

week (butt & gut/kickboxing/step) and you're automatically cross- trained. When you just do what you're good at, like tennis or running, you set yourself up for overuse injuries. Knee surgeries and artificial hipsters, anyone? Your body works harder at a new thing and cross training can blast you out of a plateau. It's kind of like the wife who knows all her husband's jokes—he gets no response. Check shape.com, Netsweat, and prevention.com for online support groups and new ideas. The *Curves* circuit training is efficient, alternating cardio with resistance; just be sure you're comfortable with the financial commitment and being in that same setting for one to three years. Enjoy nature, join a team, enjoy walking time alone; do whatever it takes.

- **Add some jumping (some impact) to your routines** if you are in fairly good shape and don't have knee or back pain. In the 80's, we started low impact aerobics to save our joints, but it turns out that some vertical jumping and jumping jacks can really help increase and maintain bone density.
- First add frequency (days/week), then duration (minutes or steps on a pedometer), then intensity (jog, speed, hills). Use Leslie Sansone's *Walk Away the Pounds Express* for in-home video walking on rainy days.

The Checklist

❏ **I. Check out the triad of tough/love trainers at your bookstore: Jim Karas, *Flip the Switch*; Bob Greene, *Get With the Program*; and Jorge Cruise, *8 Minutes in the Morning*.** Each book has commonsense advice about eating and exercise, inspiration, success stories, and suggested exercise regimens. Buy one of these books, read it, and use the exercise logs, food diaries, and guided explorations of your emotional eating. You will be experiencing the finest personal training for pennies a day!

❏ **2.** New hope for exercisers sidelined by joint pain—QuickFlex softgels or cream, fatty acid esters shown to increase flexibility and reduce pain in a study reported in the Journal of Rheumatology. High-gradient, high-gauss magnet therapy by Magna Bloc also targets pain effectively. QuickFlex and Magna Bloc are available on quixtar.com.

❏ **3.** If you're buying home equipment, check Consumer Reports and try before you buy. **Best long-haul cardio investment—a treadmill in front of the TV.** Good ones can be had for around $700 and up, but pay over $1,000 if someone will run on it or a walker weighs over 220 lbs. Recumbent bikes are good if you want to read or talk on the phone while cycling. Home ellipticals are OK, but not as good as the health club models, and don't have the programs and variable inclines of a treadmill. If you live in a warm climate, I wouldn't bother with a cardio machine. Forget ab gadgets — buy exercise tubing, a bench, some weights, and a ball for about 150 bucks. You can tape exercise shows from television, borrow videos from the library, or invest in a few excellent videos by The Firm, available at Wal-Mart or on collagevideo.com.

❑ **4.** Did you know there's as much as 80 lbs of pressure on your breasts when you exercise, stretching supporting ligaments permanently? An Australian study found 25% better support with a sports bra than a regular bra; I like the Shock Absorber, whose motto is "only the ball should bounce."

❑ **5.** A half hour before exercise, increase blood flow and stamina with ginkgo and Siberian ginseng (eleuthero), combined in one supplement in Nutrilite's Siberian EnerG. A dose of vitamin E can ease soreness for weekend warriors who've overdone it. Forget ephedra!

❑ **6.** For home strength training, try The Firm *Maximum Body Shaping* and Tamilee Web's *I Want Those Arms/I Want Those Buns. Sean O'Malley's Guided Workout* audio CD is like having a personal trainer pushing you, and Shape music CD's keep your cardio pumping with original artists; *Shape Walk 3* and *Cardio 2 & 4* are faves. I love Brian Kest's Power Yoga Videos—just watching this hunk speeds up your heart rate! Collagevideo.com is a super source for exercise videos.

❑ **7.** When you sit on an exercise ball, your thighs should be parallel with the floor—most people buy one that's too small. If you're over 5'7" tall, buy a 65-cm ball; 5' to 5'7", use a 55-cm; and if you're under 5', try 45-centimeter. Gin Miller's *Flexaball Workout* is a great bargain for beginners and her *Xtreme Strength Ball Workout* is killer. The Zone *Body Sculpt Big Ball Workout* and *QuickFIX Stability Ball Workout* are also challenging.

The Checkup from the Neck Up

❏ Each step and each repetition brings me closer to a healthy body.

❏ I'm already experiencing the benefits of breathing deeply, moving my body, quieting my mind, feeling light, loose, strong and stretched.

❏ I don't have to do things perfectly—the minute I move, I succeed.

❏ The pride lasts longer than the pain; I'll forget the inconvenience and annoyances of starting this program when my strength and endurance open new worlds for me.

❏ Instead of focusing on the size and shape of my body, I'm thrilled about the size of my attitude, confidence, and stress-free mind!

5.

Is Your Life Worth 30 Minutes a Day?
Answer Yes and Get Consistent!

> *"…I must admit that I am still not fond of sweating. In fact, I dislike it about as much as filling out income tax forms or standing in line at the Department of Motor Vehicles. But I'm used to it. About three times a week, I make sure I sweat. I do not look forward to it, but it's great when it's over…The jocks and I both get firmer thighs and happier brain chemicals. If they're firmer than I am, good for them. I know they're no happier."*
>
> <u>Fit from Within,</u> **Victoria Moran**

When you know that a program of exercise and healthy foods is the top thing you can do for your health, why don't you change? You know it slashes your risk of heart disease, all kinds of cancer, PMS, depression, Alzheimer's, arthritis, and osteoporosis. Intellectually, emotionally, and from personal experience, you are absolutely sure that adopting these behaviors would change your life for the better. So what's holding you back?

"I hate analyzing that emotional stuff."

Yeah, I do too, but something powerful is keeping you from doing what you want to do. You've tried all the ab-buster pills and machines, the lunch-in-a-can, and the no-carb diet. I hope you're convinced that stuff is junque (that's junk that costs a lot) and it's not coming to your rescue. Vegetables, healthy fats, lean protein, whole grains, and regular exercise are the answer – and you know it! When you've had a tough week, why do you order the Burger Basket with free sundae instead of a salad and a piece of fish? Why do you zone out in front of the TV instead of walking the dog and pumping some iron? The problem must be in your brain and the way you think about eating, exercise, and yourself.

Are you stepping in FOOPO?

In Chapter 1, I talk about the idea that everything is caused by either fear or love. **Are you afraid of something and do you love yourself enough to make exercise and diet a priority?** Do you suffer from FOF, FOOPO, or FOS—fear of failure, fear of other people's opinions, or fear of success? Does your inner critic witness your previous failures and tell you you'll fail again? Reading this passage, do you hear a low buzz in the back of your mind—"Yeah, I know I should exercise, I've tried and quit a million times, yada yada yada yada…"? Stop doing that! Don't give in to the yadayada! Answer it with "Yes, I'm succeeding and persisting at this exercise thing." Just as you do in meditation, you must center yourself. Think "That's OK, I'll come back to moving forward." Quiet those voices, putting one self-caring thought in front of the other like footsteps.

Instead of believing you're setting a good example, do you fear that others will think your healthy cooking and weight training is "selfish"—just about the scariest insult you can throw at a woman? Will success cause people to look more closely at you, be jealous of you, or try to bring you back to their level? Those who harvest crabs know you can't keep one in the basket, but if you put a bunch of them in there, the bottom ones pull the climbers back in. Even people who love you may fear that you'll pull away after big changes. Have you noticed that just when you start seeing results, other things in your life seem more "urgent", you fall back into your comfort zone, and you lose your forward momentum?

These are the attitude diseases that stem from a feeling of unworthiness—the core belief that you don't really deserve success and happiness. For every little girl who was told she was "a bad girl," "not as good as your sister," "the chubby one who's not athletic," "the kid who won't amount to much"— there's a woman who still believes these lies. You may consciously feel you deserve to be happy and healthy, but unconsciously feel the opposite.

The best way to defeat that garbage? Put a picture of yourself on the frig from a time when you really liked your body—from high school, your wedding, whatever. Hang the cool pair of jeans from when you had a happy body image in a prominent place. Shine the bright light of recognition on the lies you believe about yourself by writing an essay about why you *don't* deserve to be happy and healthy and the excuses you've heard yourself use to justify why you *don't* exercise and eat healthier foods. I'm not usually in favor of speaking or writing negatives, but just this once you have to recognize your own negative self-talk and mind games. Really wallow in it, and remember times when you were achieving your goals and you just…stopped. How did you explain it to yourself? You'll be amazed at how recognizing your own con job will keep you from repeating it the next time! It all looks so stupid, just sitting there in black and white.

I don't have time. **Do you watch television**, surf the Internet, waste time on the phone or reading magazines? Could you get up earlier or work out after work? Time spent exercising = time *not* spent in doctor's offices, having no energy, picking up prescriptions, and dealing with illness.

I love to eat. **Who doesn't?** Healthy people enjoy their food, but they're on a budget calories in are low, strength training and cardio are high. Can you eat half?

My family won't eat that stuff. **Are you doing them a favor** by not making gradual changes toward good health? Do you really want them to get to the point of desperation you're at?

I want to relax. **I want to have a life.** Exercise does more to clear your head and make you feel less anxious than any activity. Strength training ensures that you'll be able to climb into the boat, take the trip, learn scuba diving, and enjoy the kids and the grandkids. Cut-up veggies and salad stuff, frozen veggies, healthy cereal, fruit and protein smoothies, and chicken breasts and fish are easy and cheap. The pay-off in a high-quality life is priceless.

I don't have the energy. The person saying this is often depressed and feels powerless for various reasons. Exercise, healthy food, adequate sleep and happy relationships *create* energy. Something else is missing.

It's boring and I'm not making progress. If you're bored and punching the fitness clock, do something different, tougher, more fun or with a friend. **If all you're doing is *not* gaining weight, you're still ahead of the crowd!**

It's so hard for women. Yes, menstrual periods, childbirth, hormone changes, and less muscle mass and testosterone make it harder for women and easier for men to be lean. So what? We can't change it, we just have to deal with it.

My family makes me fat. If you heard, "She's a big girl,"

"*You* can't wear an outfit like that," "Our family tends to be big," and "Just this once. Have some" all your life, or comments were constantly made about what you ate, or your mother was constantly dieting, then yes, your family was part of your problem. But now that we know that, can we deprogram and move on? **Your gene pool does not determine your jean size!**

It's just too late. 90-year-olds who strength-trained three times a week showed a 174% increase in strength. It's too late for what? As you age, you will lose strength faster than a younger person; another reason to continue to spin those Vitamin X plates.

I'm on vacation. It's a holiday. Exercise will minimize the damage from those margarita's, midnight buffets, holiday cookies, etc.

Hey, I could just drop dead like John Ritter—I might as well live it up! Yes, you could be the one in thousands who have an unknown heart defect or brain aneurysm and drop dead even though you exercise like a fiend. But do you want to bet the quality of your life on that? The essence of "The John Ritter Factor" is—do appropriate self-care, enjoy your family and your life, and always have the next project on the drawing board!

People often ask "How much exercise is enough?"

These same people talk about health, weight loss, and fitness as if it were all the same program. Certainly, each is on the road to the other and they're all positive, but your motivation and the intensity of your program are different if you've had a heart attack than if you want to look good for your 25th high school reunion. The U.S. Surgeon General reported that you could reap "significant health benefits" from 30 minutes of moderate activity most days of the week. Beat stroke, diabetes, and heart disease in a couple of hours a week, with walking and some push-ups and sit-ups. Jorge Cruise shows you how to do it optimally with just 8 *Minutes in the Morning.*

We've already talked about weight loss—80% food choices and 20% (about 5 hours a week) exercise. Then there's fitness. I've known women who are 20 or 30 pounds overweight, yet they're very fit and strong. I've known thin, flabby women and robust middle-of-the-roaders. You may choose a couple of hours a week for health or twice that for fitness, and *that's* OK! To me, exercise is like a drug, a high, a release. I love to sweat, I can't live without it. I get off track at times, and I don't see the gains I'd like to, I enjoy a crazy amount of food at a great restaurant, but I never quit. I feel blessed that life hasn't beaten this attitude out of me, and I know that if you'd only start on the road, the rewards would keep *you* going.

The Checklist—(Other Vitamin X Attitudes:)

❑ **I. If you really want it, you'll find the time.** Whether it's health, weight loss, or fitness, you'll do it if you make it a priority. On Sunday nights, write your workouts in your calendar—in pen.

❑ **2. Keep moving and visualize victory.** Sometimes you wonder if you're doing the right thing, if you could be more effective, if it's worth it; this is fatigue and doubt talking. Imagine the fatigue flying out of your body, picture a magical coolant coursing through your body, or visualize an anti-gravity lotion keeping you light and loose. Just keep going and grab some expertise where you can. If you're looking, it will present itself.

❏ **3. The difference between a rut and a grave is the dirt on your face.** If you just keep walking the same walk, taking the same step class, and running with no goal, you see no improvement and diminishing returns. In exercise, as in life, you've got to get out of your comfort zone and kick it up a notch.

❏ **4. Tap in to the power of the team.** Whether it's a trainer, a walking/running buddy, or a familiar instructor and classmates, someone else's pace and perspective makes a huge difference. Even a friend cheering you on makes your program a team effort. Work through differences in ability; a rising tide raises all ships.

❏ **5. Avoid Boomeritis and Quick-Fix-Me-Itis.** Boomeritis is prevalent among runners and triathletes; they insist on performance breakthroughs each year. A personal best for each year is a better goal. Just don't let a really old chick beat you! Those who go to multiple doctors and try multiple therapies without giving any of them time to work mean well, but they've got to have a little patience. That tic in your shoulder will go away eventually if you baby it and stretch it but keep moving in a different way.

❏ **6. Accept what you got from your Grandma.** Bubble butt. Flat chest. Short legs. We used to stuff Kleenex in our bras, but now there's this pressure to pay a surgeon to sculpt our bodies. Okay, you say, I don't live on the Discovery Channel, where a big butt is a sign of fertility. But no one else, especially your man, is as critical of your body as you are. He likes your enthusiasm and the fact that you like *him*. Do what you need to do and then enjoy what you've got.

❏ **7. Make big deposits in your Health Bank Account for later.** We feel entitled to lots of fun and pleasure as we age and don't view body changes as "normal." That's good, but the fact is that nature only cares about us while we're reproducing —after that, we're on our own to delay the aging process. Don't wait until you're staring at the ceiling in Intensive Care.

❏ **8. Nothing works like work.** I don't care how positive your attitude is, if you don't get out there and do it you won't see benefits. Learn the right phrases to say back to yourself when you're making excuses, whether it's "I'm investing in myself today" or "Get your butt out and do it!"

The Checkup from the Neck Up

❏ I am persisting and succeeding at this exercise thing!

❏ The process of fitness is becoming play for me; feeling good will be the end product.

❏ When I exercise, I relax to the max – my shoulders, neck, jaw, hands, and mind are loose and limber.

❏ If 20 minutes is all the time I have, I do something because healthy moments add up.

❏ I listen to my body, I stay hydrated, I warm up and stretch.

❏ I have plenty of energy and when I take care of my body I create even more!

❏ I deserve this investment in myself and use my imagination to stay "above bored."

6.

Devour and Conquer—
Anti-Aging Food Factoids You Can Use

"A friend who is just turning forty lamented to me recently that he
was getting to the age when bodies break down. 'I think the human
body comes with a forty-year warranty,' he told me, 'and after that
*it starts to go to hell'…***What I think happens is not that the***
warranty runs out, but that the bill comes due. *That is, the*
cumulative effects of unhealthy habits and patterns of living make
themselves known for the first time, as the natural resilience of the
body inevitably begins to diminish."
—Andrew Weil, M.D., <u>8 Weeks to Optimum Health</u>

It's been surprising lately that some of the foods we thought
were out of our lives have come back. Peanut butter, nuts, and
olive oil—good fats. Eggs—the perfect protein. The tea my
kids were drinking that I called "crapple" is now an antioxidant
nectar of the gods. Dove Dark chocolate—polyphenol-rich
selenium booster.

Jean Carper and her book *Food—Your Miracle Medicine* were
ahead of the crowd with the power food trend. When she
started preaching "food pharmacy," people thought she was a

bit of a crackpot, but today the message of healing foods screams from every magazine. She writes that "The food pharmacy is as viable as the pill pharmacy, and more complex. Nobody has yet invented a 'broccoli pill' that can match eating the real thing, for example, and probably never will. A single food contains hundreds or thousands of chemicals, most unidentified, that make up each bite's varied pharmacological activity."

Tea for Thee. Basically, your health equals the health of your arteries, and tea protects arteries by relaxing them and influencing blood-clotting factors. Though green has a slight clump-busting edge over black, both are great at blocking bad cholesterol and inhibiting cancer cell growth. Building up bones, retarding tooth decay and bad breath, and speeding up metabolism and weight loss are also attributed to tea, and trials applying tea concentrates to skin lesions made them shrink. Reviews in *Health* and the *Nutrition Action Healthletter* found home-brewing bagged Lipton, Salada, and Tetley to have the most antioxidants, though even sweetened Snapple had some. The more you swish the bags around, the more nutrients you get. Overnight fridge tea, liquid concentrate, powdered, decaff using the carbon monoxide method (not ethyl acetate)—it's all good, and you can flavor it with some Concord grape juice, super antioxidant Buckwheat (dark) honey, or a slice of lemon to take the nutrition over the top. I find a few cups of tea keep me working through the late afternoon with less of a jolt or stomach upset than coffee. Mint tea is good for cramps, ginger for nausea and digestion, and chamomile tea is a sleep aid. "Red Zinger" Jamaican sorrel tea is reputed to lower blood pressure, fight skin cancer, and boost immunity.

Low-Fat Dairy does double duty. One percent non-BST milk stabilizes blood sugar by providing carbs, protein, and a little fat so you stay full longer. **Keeping the 1%** also leaves in some CLA, a fatty acid reputed to build muscle, bust carcinogens, and build immunity. Our family recently went organic with both milk and eggs, foods very affected by toxins and antibiotics. Calcium helps the body burn fat, and calcium consumers lost the most weight in several studies. Its built-in Vitamin D helps you absorb the calcium for your bones, and of course, dairy-rich yogurt has it's own anti-aging reputation. I love Dannon Light n' Fit Yogurt, Swiss Miss Fat-Free Cocoa with Calcium, and Cabot Vermont Cheddar Cheese-50% Light.

Beans, baby, beans! With potassium and magnesium that lowers blood pressure; soluble fiber to reduce cholesterol, cancer, and blood sugar; and folic acid to reduce homocysteine, beans are about the handiest health food around. Just open the can, rinse off the salty water, and sprinkle on salads, veggies, soups, and whole wheat pasta and tortillas. Cut the sodium and sugar in side-dish saucy beans by adding a can of plain, rinsed pinto beans—they still taste great, and it's less calories per serving. Get with the flavored hummus program—spicy, garlic, pesto—it's a great sub for cream cheese and zips up your dip. Soy burgers and soy milk are also in this group.

Why do we have more gas at midlife? The colon slows down, you may be lactose intolerant, and less estrogen may speed up the movement of food through the intestines—all recipes for gas disasters. Sorbitol in sugar-free products can be explosive. My family knows the reason I sometimes "wander off" while on a group excursion. Eliminate dairy and then add it back, seeing if symptoms return with the dairy. Lactaid can help, and Nutrilite Digestive Enzyme Complex or Beano with lots of water can help with the bean foods.

Out with the white stuff, in with the whole grains. Your body can't tell the difference between sugar and white bread, but heart disease, stroke, diabetes, and cancer love the stuff!

Women in the Nurses Health Study who ate the most whole grains cut their stroke risk by up to 40%. Wonder Stone Ground 100% Whole Wheat, Matthew's Whole Wheat English Muffins, Thomas' Whole Wheat Pita, sprouted wheat, cracked wheat, whole grain rye—what you can't find in the supermarket, you can find in the health food store. The first ingredient must be whole grain; just because it's brown, doesn't mean it's whole. Freeze half the loaf in a zip lock, especially if you're the only one eating it.

Go for the oat bran, All-Bran, Raisin Bran, Kashi, and the like, mixed with wheat germ, ground flaxseed, berries and bananas. Mix them with your old corn flakes, Fruit Loops, and Cheerios at first so you don't feel like you're eating twigs. How about tuna on whole wheat for breakfast, and cereal with fruit and milk as an evening snack? The protein revs your morning and the carbs help you sleep. Popcorn, whole grain couscous and pasta, and brown rice – it's a whole new world of fiber-rich flavor. The psyllium husk laxatives like Metamucil are the best fiber supplement choice, but they don't block hunger like tasting, chewing, and swallowing real food does.

Nuts to you are part of your "good monounsaturated fats" program, sprinkled on cereal, veggies, salads, and yogurt. Walnuts and almonds-with-skin are the most phytonutrient-healthy, and about nine nuts are enough for one snack. Pecans and macadamias are not in the program. I found *Prevention's* Peanut Butter Diet (prevention.com) effective; it adds about 4 tablespoons of peanut butter to foods throughout a healthy eating day. Surprisingly, commercial brands like Jiff worked about as well for the diet as nothing-added peanut butters. The satisfying spread keeps hunger away and lowers cholesterol; when you have it daily, you stop wanting to eat half the jar, believe me.

The facts on the fats—it's confusing, but important. My

young adults, growing up in the low-fat 80's, still think low-fat is automatically good—*they're* in the stone age on this one! Way back in the day, margarine was considered better than butter; then we found the trans fats (partially hydrogenated oils) in margarine were worse than the sat fat in butter, and went back to butter. Then in the 90's, we all rushed out and bought olive oil, believing only monounsaturated fat was good; now recent research shows that polys have more power to lower bad cholesterol than monos! **What seems safest right now is to cook and bake mostly with canola oil,** to balance the use of soy oil in prepared foods and restaurants. Use olive oil for salad dressing or to flavor veggies, and light use of cooking sprays is fine. A new player on the scene, Enova oil, claims that the fat it uses is burned quickly, not stored, by the body.

Scale back the full-fat mayo to the light kind; try Spectrum Canola Light to get away from more soy oil. **In your margarine or spread, go low in salt and both trans and sat-fats;** I like Smart Beat Trans Fat Free Super Light Margarine for family use. Say yes to the Take Control and Benecol Light Spread — their plant extracts lower cholesterol – but they haven't been studied enough yet for children and pregnant women. A light spritz of I Can't Believe It's Not Butter spray is handy for veggies. Choose sharp, flavorful cheeses so you can use less; cheese and white pasta are usually the culprits behind fat vegetarians. Your upper limit for sat fat is 12g/day, and one slice of premium Muenster is 7 grams.

Gettin' fishy with it is important—study after study shows very significant heart health gains from consuming fish. The list of benefits from Omega 3's and other nutrients in salmon, tuna, and other fatty fish gets longer every week, including preventing blood clots and sudden cardiac death, lowering blood pressure and triglyceride levels, and raising HDL cholesterol.

If you dislike broiling or grilling fish at home, order it when you're out and have canned salmon or tuna at home a few times a week, mixed with Walden Farms calorie-free dips. Recently there had been some concerns about mercury pollution from ocean fish—particularly shark, swordfish, and king mackerel— so I was happy to buy farm-raised fish at my market. Then a report came out about PCB's in the food given to farm-raised fish! The fish farmers are getting that under control as we speak, so eating a variety of fish like salmon, whitefish, and light tuna is fine. My desire for fish variety led me to buy my first can of boneless, skinless sardines, since I keep reading that they're packed with omega 3's. I rinsed off the soya oil, mashed it up with some flavored light GourMayo, and put it on toast. It tasted like tuna, only a little stronger and saltier. Be brave, try new fishies!

Or not. Many people just don't like fish, and **a number of clinical trials now support the benefits of fish oil pills.** Combined pills of DHA and EPA that get you between 1,000 or 2,000 mg a day is a good goal. For those who can't even stomach that or have fish allergies, ground flaxseed on your cereal should get enough omega-3's to your heart. The DHA in the new omega-3 eggs is probably not enough to really affect heart health.

The antioxidant power of berries is so impressive, doctor's are "prescribing" these little "pills" to fight many conditions of aging: maintaining night vision, reversing short term memory loss, blocking bladder problems, shrinking tumors, raising HDL, and easing pain. Organic fruits and vegetables may be even more healthful, since they're 20 to 50% higher in antioxidants. It's really all part of your drive to Eat Nine a Day, nine servings of brightly colored fruits and vegetables, but blueberries, cranberries, and raspberries are especially high in natural disease-fighters. Your cereal now has banana, ground flaxseed, and 1% milk on it, but go ahead and add some berries.

Have some Northland 27% Cranberry Juice blended with grape, peach, and six other flavors. Throw berries in your yogurt, on a salad, or in a smoothie, or just put them on a plate, drizzled with Walden Farms delicious calorie-free chocolate sauce. Berry cousin The Grape keeps getting rave reviews for heart disease and cancer prevention, with red wine serving as the possible explanation to "the French paradox"—how do they eat rich foods and stay so slim and healthy? I used to hesitate to buy expensive fruits, but now I compare them with medication and supplements and realize they're a bargain!

In Nina Shandler's wonderful book, *Estrogen: The Natural Way—Over 250 Easy and Delicious Recipes for Menopause*, **soy and flaxseed are incorporated into recipes** designed to decrease cholesterol, menopause symptoms, breast and prostate cancer, and osteoporosis risks. I chuckle when I picture Nina checking out at the supermarket with multiple containers of tofu. The teenager at the cash register was thinking, "Here comes that whack job again!" Shandler's recipes for tofu mayonnaise and dip can add those creamy substances back into your life without all the fat and calories. Her granolas are power-packed with isoflavones and lignans. Supplementing Nina's way will probably work the best, because you're **using the food factors, the whole food, rather than something extracted from soy.**

The debate over soy epitomizes our longing for natural solutions to midlife and menopause health issues. We hope that if we only add enough soy isoflavones to our diet, we will live to a heart-healthy, cancer-free old age like the Asian women we keep reading about! Soy is added to cereal and all kinds of foods, and the soy milk section of the supermarket expands weekly. A new player in the soy foods game is Ketatos, high-fiber and protein, low-carb and -calorie mashed potato substitutes. On the other hand, Asians don't generally eat soybeans in these formats. They eat *fermented* soy foods in the form of tempeh, miso, and tamari. They eat very little animal fat, tons of fish and seafood, consume less alcohol, and incorporate more exercise into their daily lives than we do. These factors could be relevant, ya' think? In addition, soy isoflavones are like estrogen and may have the same effects, so these foods and supplements are not necessarily "safer." Soy may compete with our body's own declining hormones at receptor sights. For example, women trying to get pregnant should not use soy, since it interacts with ovarian function. The use of soy supplements and powders has studies pro and con; a large study on a popular isoflavone supplement showed *no difference* in hot flashes between the placebo and the isoflavone group, yet many women swear by them.

Garlic, onions, broccoli, BroccoSprouts, spinach, collard greens, apples, papaya, prunes, dried apricots, oatmeal, red wine, citrus fruits, watermelon, tomatoes, organic eggs—there are new discoveries every day about the "pharmacy" in these foods. "If we are what we eat, I'm fast, cheap, and easy" used to describe me, but our refrigerator has been revolutionized in recent years and we all get more of the good stuff.

The Checklist

❑ I. For an anti-cancer diet, get *A Dietitian's Cancer Story*, by Diana Dyer. Here's her Super Shake: 1/3 cup silken tofu; 6 baby carrots; 1 cup fresh fruit; 1 tbsp ea wheat bran, wheat germ, and ground flaxseed; 1 cup ea calcium-fortified soy milk and orange juice.

❑ 2. How to have a whole day's calories (over 2,000) and 5 day's worth of saturated fat in one meal: prime rib,

Caesar salad, and loaded potato; fettuccini alfredo, salad w/dressing, garlic bread; Burger King double whopper w/cheese, huge fries & cola. (from *Restaurant Confidential*)

❑ **3.** Subway now has ten low-fat sandwiches, "7 Subs with 7 Grams of Fat or Less" and three "Select Subs." Wendy's Mandarin Chicken salad (1/2 dressing, skip noodles), BK Veggie Burger, and McDonald's Fruit 'n Yogurt Parfait are other good choices.

❑ **4.** A serving of raw veggies or fruit is the size of a baseball, cooked serving the size of a fist. Add up what you eat on caloriescount.org.

❑ **5.** Best "meaty" soy burgers—Flame Grilled Gardenburgers, Morningstar Farms Grillers, Roasted Garlic Boca Burgers, Veggie Patch Garlic Portobello. Spicy favorites are Dr. Praeger's Tex Mex and Morningstar Farms Spicy Black Bean.

❑ **6.** Keep a checklist on the counter: vegetables, fruits, whole grains, calcium foods, beans, nuts, fish, water, tea.

The Checkup from the Neck Up

❑ I've accepted the challenge of creating powerful new eating habits.

❑ A rising tide raises all ships, and my power-food diet benefits everyone in my house.

❑ The rainbow of fruits and vegetables I eat makes my cells celebrate and scrubs the bad stuff out of my veins.

❑ When I eat well consistently, I have faith that my body will stop craving sugar, fat, and salt and totally enjoy and prefer healthy foods.

❑ If you are what you eat, I am amazing!

7.

If You Ate Like a Monkey, You Wouldn't Need Supplements—But Do You?
Supplements, water, and sleep to take life to the next level

"Women often tell me that herbal medicine is 'more natural' and therefore safer. Herbs aren't necessarily 'gentler' or 'safer' than pharmaceutical products. For example, I have seen quite a number of patients, as well as myself, who have had allergic reactions or toxicity symptoms to herbal products...I also have patients who have had adverse reactions to prescription pharmaceuticals...no matter what the source, there is the potential for benefit as well as the possibility of an undesirable reaction."
—Elizabeth Lee Vliet, M.D., <u>Women, Weight, and Hormones</u>

Monkeys get a host of nutrients from their plant-based diet of fruits, leaves, grasses, flowers and tree bark. And of course, they get a lot of exercise swinging around on trees gathering their dinner! Women who're struggling to overthrow the pizza-based diet and get their nine plants-a-day need supplements, and they need to discover ways to make sure they take them. Remembering and feeling worthy of your self-care is half the battle. 30% of participants in a bone density study stopped taking their calcium, even though solid benefits were personally proven to them!

I've tried keeping my supplements neatly lined up in the kitchen cabinet, but that's where they stay—in the cabinet instead of in my body! Bathroom medicine chest? Too much moisture, and you forget they're in there. I use **the "basket system," a pretty open basket with all our supplements that I leave out on the counter.** Friends have duplicated this system with great success. You can stash the basket in a cabinet if you need the counter space for a party. Forget about canisters (you're cutting back on flour and sugar anyway) and cute cookie jars—taking your supplements is more important!

Associate morning and nighttime rituals with taking your supplements, keeping in mind that many are best taken with a meal. If you take a birth control pill or other medication, supplements can usually be taken at the same time. A foil or plastic pack with a dose worth of vitamins is very luxurious and great for work or travel, and saves you opening and closing the bottles—hire your teen to put each dose in a tiny zip lock bag. Nutrilite XX blister strips and Leading Edge Heart Packs are prepackaged and ready to go where you go. I don't care for plastic containers with compartments, because in my experience too much air gets to the supplements and degrades them.

The consequences of not taking your supplements consistently can be far-reaching. I've noticed a pattern—

- In your early forties, you start throwing down supplements without changing your crazy lifestyle. You don't see results 'cause you're not consistent.

- When you hit 45 or so, you start making some weak attempts at lifestyle changes and continue to take even more supplements "when you remember."
- At 50 or 55, an acquaintance your age dies suddenly, and you realize your health is not a game. Frightened, you dump all your supplements and start taking every prescription drug you can get your hands on. Not the most effective behavior, is it?

There can be *too much* of a good thing in individual nutrients like Vitamins A, D, and E, so recently the Food and Nutrition Board established the (UL) upper intake level: the maximum amount of a vitamin or mineral that's safe on a long term daily basis. *Prevention* magazine has these UL's on its web site roundup of the perfect multivitamin, but remember that **the figure includes the total amount from food *and* supplements.** A Harvard study showed that postmenopausal women taking 5,000 IU of Vitamin A (that's the cheap kind that's *not* from beta carotene) had double the risk of hip fracture, so make sure your supplement has beta carotene, not retinol. Too much Vitamin E could lead to internal bleeding and too much Vitamin D included in calcium supplements could be toxic.

The upper level for calcium is 2,500 mg (with 1,200 recommended). You're over that at breakfast if you take a multi and a calcium supplement (1,000 mg) and three foods fortified with calcium: orange juice (350 mg), cereal (1,000 mg), and milk (500mg). Luckily (?), your body only absorbs about 35% of the calcium you take in. Taking the antibiotic Cipro with calcium-enriched orange juice reduces the drug's absorption by 40%.

Why all the fuss? Should you bet your health on supplements? Should you gamble that the perfect combination of pills will win you the lottery of perfect health? No, you've got to eat a great diet, but everyone from the surgeon general to Harvard researchers to your mama recommends at least one multivitamin that includes calcium, folic acid, and Vitamins D, B6, & B12 daily to prevent chronic disease.

The old apple, she ain't what she used to be.

Barely 10% of us eat enough plant food and our bodies absorb fewer nutrients as we age. Most foods are not eaten fresh. In a Canadian study comparing government food tables from 1951 with those from 1999, levels of calcium, vitamins A & C, and iron had dropped as much as 80% in broccoli, potatoes, and apples. High-yield farming strategies, long-haul trucking, and food storage methods contribute to the depletion of vitamins and minerals in the food supply. In addition, the phytonutrients and associated food factors are depleted, and we're just beginning to understand how plant chemicals like lycopene, ellagic acid, and quercetin help the body prevent disease. Medical authorities now agree that everyone needs at least a multivitamin to address the deficits in our foods.

Is the supplement what it says it is? Answering this question is important for your health and your wallet. A 2003 study of Echinacea preparations found ingredients varied widely and that 10% of the 59 products tested had no measurable Echinacea at all! One manufacturer touted their calcium by citing a study that used only eleven patients for four weeks; the absorption difference was so small it was not significant, but they used it anyway.

But I haven't worried about what's in my supplements since I found Nutrilite in 1979, and my respect for their quality has grown with each passing year. I've been to their farm in California, and their organic farming methods border on the fanatical, using compost instead of chemical fertilizers and ladybugs instead of chemicals to kill pests. They process the fruit and plant concentrates within four hours of picking, to preserve their nutritional value and phytonutrients. Nutrilite formulates great complementary blends—E with natural selenium, ginkgo biloba with DHA, acerola C with a bioflavonoid concentrate—that make the supplements better absorbed and more effective in the body. Most glucosamine comes from the shells of shrimp that are grown on farms, raised in close quarters and treated with antibiotics; Nutrilite harvests shrimp from the pristine North Atlantic Ocean. A recent study revealed that people who took CoQ10 in an oil-based softgel showed higher levels of the enzyme in their blood. Guess what? My newest batch of Nutrilite CoEnzymeQ10 showed up in a rice bran-oil softgel. Yes, they're more expensive than supermarket brands, but available at a discount member price on Quixtar.com. Yes, the big warehouse brands and health food store lines are good products, but I've decided to go first class with Nutrilite.

PMS and perimenopause supplements are big business, and every doctor and nutritionist seems to have their favorites. Experts seem united on the value of ground **flaxseed** or flaxseed oil; **GLA from evening primrose** and borage oil; and fatty fish or **fish oil** supplements. They may heal your heart and general health while mending your PMS symptoms, so you can't miss with these. Barlean's flaxseed oils—in the refrigerated section at markets and health food stores—are excellent, and they make a special "Essential Woman Healing Oil" with four kinds of fatty acids, lignans, and other nutrients. You can throw a tablespoon in yogurt, oatmeal, or a protein drink each morning. Getting your EPA's and DHA's from eating salmon and other fatty fish is optimal, but companies like Quixtar's Ocean Essentials, Costco's Kirkland Signature, and Sam's Club Member's Mark make high-quality fish oil and GLA supplements you should add to your routine. To avoid fish burps, freeze them.

Homeopathy is a natural way to combat symptoms without estrogen-like substances. It uses the science of "like heals like," and common peri- and menopause ingredients include damiana, lechesis, sepia, salvia, and pulsatilla. Go to iVillage Market for an excellent selection of Cayor homeopathic products. Find a practitioner through homeopathic.org.

I have to be honest and report that double-blind, placebo-controlled studies of peri- and menopause herbals have been disappointing. In addition, a recent small study found more aggressive tumor growth in mice given black cohosh. If you want to address your symptoms with herbals, the two to start with are chasteberry (also called **vitex**) and **dong quai.** You must take these and all herbals consistently for three months to see if they're working. Together with Vitamin E, B6, and calcium with magnesium, they could alleviate the tough periods, irritability, flashes, and dark moods. Standardized versions of each abound, or you can use combos like Nutrilite PriMroSe Plus, or iVillage's PMS Peacemaker.

Beat the sweats. Black cohosh, red clover, and soy are used as your periods taper off, closer to and during menopause. These products have estrogen-like effects, so if you fear estrogen, think twice before using them. Remifemin is the well-known black cohosh supplement, and Emerita's Menopause Plus Formula blends it with red clover, while Nutrilite's Black Cohosh and Soy adds soy protein, isoflavones, and bioflavonoid. There are additional thoughts about soy in Chapter 6. Enzymatic Therapy's AM/PM product combines black cohosh with ginseng and green tea for daytime energy, and adds valerian and hops to the black cohosh in the evening for sleep. When using combined products, make sure the potency is comparable to the stand-alone versions. Promensil (red clover) has 40 mg of four isoflavones in a once-a-day pill that some find effective for night sweats and other symptoms, though study results showed no benefit over placebo. A Revival soy shake at lunch—with a high dose of 160 mgs of isoflavones in one shot—ends night sweats for many women. Taken at dinner, a 200 mg time-release B6 may stop those 4 a.m. sweats. These herbals and phytoestrogens claim to boost or balance hormones, or you can attack the symptoms: gingko and ginseng for clarity and energy; passionflower and valerian for anxiety and sleep. Don't do the "more is better" thing and take everything in sight; many herbals take months to show benefits.

Put some glide in your stride with glucosamine—there are some good studies to support the use of this supplement. Some girlfriends and I were laughing recently about getting out of the car after a long ride and walking stiffly, like a weeble. Ibuprofen and naproxen help, perhaps as well or better than prescription drugs Celebrex and Vioxx, but you can't plump up cartilage with these. Glucosamine gets to the source of the problem when it stimulates the cartilage, repairs the collagen, and supports the joints you pounded running or taking high impact aerobics back in the 80's. There is some controversy about glucosamine sulfate versus glucosamine HCI and about including chondroitin in the mix, since its molecule may be too large to be absorbed and your body usually makes all the chondroitin you need. Nutritilite and iVillage have glucosamine HCI helped along by boswellia, while Wal-Mart's Spring Valley has a double strength version of glucosamine sulfate with chondroitin. SAM-e and MSM may help soothe joints, and your multi, B vitamins, GLA, and fish oil also build connective tissue.

Those healthy omega-3 fats play a role in **boosting mood and busting depression**, which is one more of many reasons

to get those EPA's and DHA's. SAM-e is a faster-acting mood
and joint supplement, available at Costco and Sam's Club but
still quite expensive. Though St John's Wort tested poorly for
major depression, it's still thought to be effective for mild to
moderate cases of the blues. It should not be used by those
taking birth control pills. Studies have largely given the
thumbs down on melatonin and kava; sleep aid valerian and
chill-pill passionflower seem to be better tolerated. If you
drink alcohol or take statin drugs or antidepressants, consider
taking milk thistle; Nature's Way Thisilyn is made by the
same German company used in European research, but
Nutrilite's version contains Siliphos, a form of silymarin that's
proven to be more potent and easily absorbed. Statin-takers
should also supplement CoQ10, but more on heart
supplements in Chapter 25.

   **Memory and mind power are all about blood flow to the
brain**, so exercise, a nutrient-rich diet, and normal blood
pressure are the first line of defense for a blooming brain.
Ginkgo biloba has some success in tests for mental sharpness,
and Ginkgold and Ginkoba are the brands identical to the
ones used in government testing in Germany. Energy-
boosting ginseng brings oxygen to *all* the tissues of the body
(brain, muscles, genitals, you name it) and Siberian EnerG
with Ginkgo Biloba from Nutrilite may boost mental *and*
physical endurance. The Russian Olympic teams admit to
using Siberian ginseng to increase performance and reduce
muscle soreness. Watch for higher blood pressure or
palpitations on ginseng. Energy drink "XS" uses ginseng,
vitamin B, and other adaptogens, while Red Bull contains the
amino acid taurine and sugar; both contain caffeine.

   Garlic is the most popular of all supplements, both for
immunity and lowering blood pressure and cholesterol, and

it's a good example of why to buy quality. ConsumerLab.com tested fourteen varieties of garlic, and active-ingredient allicin levels *varied from as little as 400 mcg to 6,500 mcg!* I take a "tickle cocktail" of garlic, natural C, and Echinacea when I feel a cold or flu coming on. Newer immunity supplements (great for traveling among foreign "bugs") include maitake and astragalus, which have the advantage of being effective for everyday use versus Echinacea, which is only recommended for occasional use.

When you're disappointed in the world and your place in it, it's hard to motivate yourself to keep up with your supplements. During down times, my eating, exercising, and general self-care hit the skids. Listen to what you're saying to yourself when you procrastinate. "Why bother? It doesn't make a difference. I don't have time." Basically the theme is that you are not worth it. Come back at yourself with a positive statement about your worth and your future. Take your supplements with a big glass of water.

Hey, speaking of water—**what kind of water are you "supplementing" your body with?** Nine to twelve cups a day keeps your energy level up and reduces cancer risk by flushing toxins and waste from the body. Women in a large 2002 study had a 40% lower risk of fatal heart attack if they drank at least five glasses of water a day. Top-rated bottled waters are Dannon, Arrowhead, Evian, Dasani, and Poland Spring. Pitcher-type purifiers work well if you can't install a filter. The ultimate answer is to use an under sink carbon filter with a faucet next to the sink for your own water, starting with Kenmore filters from Sears. GE makes a good filter, and Culligan products can be used longer before changing the filter. These systems "treat" water, removing a percentage of sediments, bacteria, viruses, and cysts.

The eSpring system from Quixtar.com actually "purifies" the water, taking 99.95% of these substances out of the water using both the carbon filter and a UV light. The eSpring filter usually lasts a family of six a year or more, beeps when it needs to be changed, and changes like a breeze. Aquacheck Labs or Hometest offer homeowner water quality test kits online.

Sleep is cheap—have you tried supplementing that?

Life runs more smoothly when you've had enough sleep. First of all, have you noticed *how much less you eat* if you go to bed early? The Chunky Monkey's not calling to you if you're already asleep. Your face looks extra puffy and wrinkly when you haven't had enough sleep. And lack of sleep leads to inflammation of the arteries which leads to heart disease—so *just do it* and get some sleep! You will find you've gained more productive, creative, focused hours in your day when you just make this one change!

Those who say they need to "watch TV to unwind" should try nodding off while reading a book in bed to test how much they "need" TV time. Practice the "sleep basics"—have a regular waking and sleeping time; cut off the caffeine; blow off the intense take-home work and TV shows; turn the clock around so you can't keep checking it; and have a cool room and a sleepy, carby snack like cereal before bed. Beyond that, try sleep deprivation – if you keep waking up at 2 a.m. and tossing and turning, take no naps and stay out of bed until seven hours before you have to wake up. No exceptions! In 4 to 6 weeks, you'll find you're sleeping through the night.

Your place or mine, baby? As the waistline expands at midlife, the volume of the snoring usually does too. There's a contest to see who can get to sleep first to avoid listening to the thunder. Alcohol and overweight make snoring much worse. The first line of defense is the tennis ball sown into the pajama top, keeping the snorer on their side. Snoring on the back is the loudest and has the strongest baseline. The snoring sprays like homeopathic SnoreStop, spritzed on the back of the throat before bed, and the Breathe Right strips do work if used regularly. They seem to cut down on the buzz saw vibrato of the snore, leaving just the loud breathing part. If there's breath-holding while snoring, it's time to go to a sleep clinic.

One answer to sleep impaired by your partner's snoring is separate sleeping rooms, facilitated when kids leave home. Are you horrified? If you've tried all the snoring remedies and the noise is still setting decibel records, having your own space may spice up your marriage by putting some mystery (and sleep) back into the relationship. Don't all the better-sex guides tell you to change locations to avoid boredom anyway?

Scott and I have the 'separate blanket' compromise (we both snore), so we can easily snore in different directions without tugging on the covers. We use quilts with flannel duvet covers in the winter, cotton covers in the summer. They get folded up and slid under the bed on plastic sleds during the day. Hey, just because your mother used the old top sheet/blanket configuration doesn't mean you have to! The duvets go in the wash just like the top sheet. Yes, a pretty cover and decorative pillows go on the bed during the day, though that's one of the things my mother did I swore I'd never do. Even if no one sees it but me, I still like it.

The Checklist

❏ I. Don't even think about using the weight-loss herbal ephedra, also known as ma huang. If high-profile athletes drop dead from it, why would a normal, puny specimen like you consider it? The new incarnation of this junque is bitter orange, with the same cardiac implications. It's a case of SCDD—same crap, different day.

❏ 2. Migraines generally get less severe after 50, which is small comfort if they're plaguing you now. Magnesium (6 to 800 mg), or 400 mg of B2 (riboflavin) can help, with higher doses under a doctor's supervision. The herbal feverfew and cutting MSG, nitrites, caffeine, aspartame (Equal), tyramine foods like aged cheeses, chocolate, and booze are worth a try.

❏ 3. CLA (conjugated linoleic acid) is interesting on a number of fronts. It reduces body fat by increasing muscle mass, has anti-cancer and immune properties, and may lower blood pressure. Take about 3g a day from Natrol, Nutrilite, or TwinLab over six months to see a result.

❏ 4. Taper your supplements down to multi and calcium before surgery. There are too many other variables to deal with, and your surgeon may not be aware of blood-thinning and other properties that could interact.

Supplements are powerful and you deserve the right ones in the right amounts!

8.

That was very 9/10 of you!
Stay on the high road with a continuous positive program of vision and laughter.

*"My version of Psalm 23's second line would read, The Lord is my shepherd; I shall **often** want. I shall yearn, I shall long, I shall aspire…If there are empty spaces in your life, dreams that never came true, people who were once there but are gone now, the purpose of those empty spaces is not to frustrate you or to brand you as a loser. The empty spaces may be there to give you room to grow, to dream, to yearn, and to teach you to appreciate what you have because it may not have been there yesterday and may not be there tomorrow."*
—**Harold S. Kushner**, <u>The Lord Is My Shepherd</u>

On September 11th, so many of us learned—for the 1st time or the 50th—what is really important about life. We felt it in the gut when we saw people searching, showing the pictures of their loved ones over and over, to any one who would stop long enough to look at them. Our hearts went out to the widow in the front row at the memorial service. Her children sat stiffly next to her in their ties and dresses purchased for happier

occasions. Blood donors lined up and money flowed in to the
Red Cross and other relief funds. Strangers looked each other
in the eye for the first time, recognizing the humanity and
shared experience of every person on the planet.

Recently, though, you may have seen someone slip into a
parking spot without yielding to the elderly couple patiently
waiting for it. The grateful tolerance you felt for your
husband's couch-napping tendencies may have once again
reverted to September 10th levels of irritation. What was it
about those television images that moved us to a higher level,
and how can we get there and stay there?

Can you tell me how to get to the High Road?

Acceptance and forgiveness of yourself and others is a day-
by-day task. When your mother blurts out an unkind remark
and your flighty friend cancels for the umpteenth time, who is
there to remind you to let these things bounce off your thick
skin and remember how closely you hold these people in your
heart? Seize the best and forget the rest is a great midlife
motto, but in the everyday world, we need reminding.

Both psychologists and clergy believe you must be in an
**automatic and ever-present positive self-improvement
program. It must be an integral part of your life**, like eating,
sleeping and exercising. Getting your words and thoughts
under control is covered in Chapter 2. If you're a reader like
me, go to a mega book store and make a list of all the uplifting
self-improvement books you'd like to read. A bible study or
women's volunteer group are obvious places to look, or you can
form an investment, book, professional, "after work" or "lunch
out" group of like-minded women who meet regularly. Cover
your frig with your favorite sayings and keep the positive music
or books-on-tape playing.

Many people—wounded by life but determined to stay on the high road—have been privileged to be part of a support group, where you are helping others and they are helping you. If your partner won't attend, set the example and go yourself. In Harold Kushner's book, *How Good Do We Have to Be?*, he pinpoints the strength of a support group where you'd find "...the redeeming knowledge that other people—nice, honorable, attractive people—were struggling with the same demons you were, and that you could do for each other what each of you had not been able to do for yourself.."

How about being a joy junkie? It has tangible health benefits, as in the Proverbs quote "A merry heart does good, like medicine, but a broken spirit dries the bones." Kids are the experts on a merry heart, since they laugh or smile about 300 times a day; adults laugh or smile only 8 to 15 times a day. You have to laugh when you hear a child's musical giggle; it's infectious! Don't you love to spend time with anyone—child or adult— who makes you see the funny side of things? Scott's grandfather George never owned anything or had a dime in the bank, but because he laughed at everything and enjoyed life, everyone loved him. You can resolve to make funny things happen or be the one who laughs the hardest, whatever works for you.

In a 1996 experiment that investigated pain relief, post-surgical patients were found to require lower doses of analgesics when they watched funny movies than when they watched serious films. **Take a funny movie like a pill, whether you need it or not.** Out-of-control laughter is like jogging for your system, massaging your insides, exercising your face, increasing blood flow and circulation, stimulating the immune system, and even fighting disease. If you've ever fallen and then laughed at how stupid you look, you know how laughter chases pain. Don't let all your good humor be the kind that comes on an ice cream stick.

Sometimes, Girls Just Wanna Have Fun!

Serious talk and introspection is not a prerequisite for self-improvement. Humor and fun help us transcend our troubles, and lift us up above fear and disappointment. Having the joke of the day delivered to your computer can protect you from uncertainty and pop the cork on your anger. Funny books in the bathroom like *Rules for Aging, Cheap Psychological Tricks*, or any of cartoonist Lyn Johnston's *For Better or Worse* books give you a quick dose of Vitamin H(umor) with your tank time.

An earned privilege of being over 40 is the right to be cranky and contrary once in a while. If you want to hurt yourself laughing at the Queen of Contrary Advice, pick up *The Sweet Potato Queen's Book of Love* or author Jill Conner Browne's latest, *The Sweet Potato Queens' Big-Ass Cookbook and Financial Planner*. With recipes for "Fat Mama's Knock-You-Naked Margaritas" and "Whatchamacallit Chicken," southern belle Browne reveals her unique perspectives on love, life, and men. Her take on everything from second careers, to strokes, to the magic words that make men do whatever you want provide a hilarious alternative to all the goody-two-shoes advice you're getting in *this* book.

Leave a legacy of laughter.

If you have children at home, throw yourself into it! Make the most of every holiday, go nuts over birthday parties, be there for every choral concert, and plan family vacations that create the legends of the future. Show them that life is tremendous and it's really worth living! Have no regrets about missing *anything* and create a model for them to follow when raising their children, a reference library of laughter that will serve them well as fun-loving spouses and parents. **They won't remember how much money was spent for gifts; they'll**

remember fun family times and how you made them a priority.

I went to a bridal shower recently, and I was struck by the smiles and infectious laughter of the bride, her sister, her mother, her grandmother, her aunt, and her aunt's daughter. They seemed determined to have the most fun of anyone at the party, and the room was lit by their enthusiasm. What will your legacy be? Will you pass on the torch of living life to its fullest? Will your children be quick to volunteer, quick to smile, quick to laugh at themselves? Have you taught them how to make a life? Have you lifted your sisters with your refusal to hold a grudge and your insistence on living on purpose, instead of accepting the leftovers life leaves behind? Do you interpret your blunders as shameful or as lessons? Will the stiff, judgmental people feel lighter with you, in spite of themselves?

Whether it's bunko or bowling, a silly hat or a clown nose, remember that **getting old isn't a reason to stop playing; stopping playing is the reason we get old.** Put on a clown nose to get an upgrade from the harried airline clerk. Our family collects talking toys like an ape singing "Wild Thing," interactive jokesters from *Monster's Inc.*, and a pair of roaring giant fists from *The Hulk.* We have a big box of funny hats, Groucho glasses, and other crazy get ups. You can't be mad at a bald guy in a Carmen Miranda hat.

Making good choices always goes back to the old sowing and reaping principle. Sowing the right actions reaps peace. That's it—period.

Life is simpler when you realize that you will reap what you sow. When choices are made to keep a certain image alive, life can get complicated trying to figure out which version of the truth you told to whom. Should you tell about your friend's divorce settlement, even though she asked you not to? If you're single, should you invite over that married guy whose wife "doesn't understand him," even though he still lives with her and their children? Is it OK to keep that item you borrowed, "because they're so wealthy they'll never miss it?"

Bad choices I've made give me a queasy stomach every time I think about them, and the good ones have blossomed and sent out more roots, shoots, and flowers then I could ever have imagined. Want to see the fruit of bad choices? Check out Maury, Jenny Jones, Jerry Springer, and the rest of the "if it feels good, I do it, whether it hurts people or not" crowd.

Am I a swingin' chick, or a mood-swingin' chick?

You wouldn't seek out a plumber to do brain surgery, would you? That's why your sister who's been divorced twice may not be the best person to advise you on the troubles you and your husband are having, right? When you just can't seem to climb out of bad feelings, it may be time to go to a professional. There's nothing they haven't heard, and because of their broad experience, they have a good idea what works and what doesn't in solving emotional troubles. Often, you must reassure your partner that seeking therapy is not a sign that you can't handle problems by yourself. It's just consulting with a professional who knows the territory, like a lawyer or a mechanic. No, they won't ask you to talk about your childhood for months, or tell you what a horrible person you are; a good therapist will focus on what's happening now and how you can move forward from here. A therapist is not a referee who decides which side gets the point, but more like a coach who builds on the skills you have to build alternatives for the future.

The purpose of marriage and family counselors is obvious; the trick is to find someone who can deal with all parties. A phone chat will give you some idea of the counselor's personality, and your first visit can be considered a try-out. Start by yourself; the counselor may help you to bring your partner into the picture. Your pastor or rabbi may help you sort things out or refer you to other counseling, or a weekend retreat sponsored by a religious organization may help your partner see that the issues you're facing are shared by others. (Women already know this because of our vast "sharing network.") Psychologists are another option, and your insurance may help to pay if your troubles are affecting your sleep, your appetite, or other aspects of your health. If you agree on a certain number of visits, they will respect that as much as they can.

Psychiatrists are medical doctors who can prescribe medications for depression and other problems, and you can go to them for the entire course of care or be referred for a few sessions, to determine if medication is appropriate and what kind would be best. **Don't feel like medication for depression or anxiety is a crutch, and it would be better if you "gut it out." The new scientific thinking is that emotions may trigger chemical changes in the brain, and that's why you may need medication and counseling to make a comeback.** Paxil is reported to have the least effect on heart rate, Prozac and Zoloft may help with PMS, and Wellbutrin is said to have the fewest sexual side effects, a problem with the SSRI type of drugs. Get your hormone levels evaluated and get on lower progestin birth control pills or estrogen replacement before taking other medications, since that can often be the cause of mood swings in midlife. Talking to a therapist **and** taking medication for a period of time can help you smooth out the wrinkles in your life before you try to fly on your own.

Left without treatment, 30 percent of depressed people will try to commit suicide. A full-blown clinical depression could

be described as "falling into a black hole," and includes some or all of these symptoms for over two weeks:
- loss of interest and pleasure in sex and enjoyable activities
- over/under eating
- too much/too little sleep
- extreme fatigue
- feelings of hopelessness, anxiety, worthlessness, guilt
- trouble concentrating

Men may manifest depression differently, turning to drugs, alcohol, extramarital sex, workaholism, risky behavior, or rage as a way of not dealing with depression and numbing the pain. Talk therapy combined with drug therapy is very successful, so there's good reason to insist your loved one get evaluated and get started on the road to a renewed appreciation of life.

The healthiest happy pill is Vitamin X!

A study at Duke University found that exercise was just as effective as the antidepressant Zoloft. **Exercise is a powerful medicine for depression and anxiety, and fortunately for you and me, the only side effect is weight loss.**

The Checklist

❏ I. You can find support groups for everything from alopecia to workaholism at sites like support-group.com, griefshare.org, and mentalhelp.net and on the major medical sites. They'll help you locate a message board or in-person group, offer toll-free support, or give you tips on starting your own group.

❏ 3. Don't tell a seriously depressed person to buck up and snap out of it, "you're going through a phase," etc. Pain is part of life, but suffering is optional, so help find a therapist who shows how to confront and change negative beliefs and manage moods. Be available for daily walks in the sunlight and be patient and help monitor the process of finding the right medication.

❏ 3. Assessments to determine if you should see a therapist are available any time on psychologytoday.org and apa.org (American Psychological Association), and the APA will get you to a local referral at 800-964-2000.

❏ 4. Always have a funny movie around like Tootsie, Some Like It Hot, Young Frankenstein, Blazing Saddles, A Fish Called Wanda, There's Something About Mary, The Nutty Professor, and Beetlejuice.

9.

Raising Kids—
Not a true-false or multiple choice test, but a never-ending essay

"When I was a boy of fourteen, my father was so ignorant I could hardly stand to have the old man around. But when I got to be twenty-one, I was astonished at how much he had learned in seven years."
—Mark Twain

Enjoying the ride, picking your spots, and talking, talking, talking is definitely what it's all about after age 11, as your kids enter their teens. Do you know their three best friends? Do you listen with acceptance to what they're concerned about, what their goals are, what they're working on at school? Have you seized opportunities to point out their strengths and share stories about your own hopes, friends, and mistakes at their age?

When my kids were growing up, I always sought out girl talk and parenting books to find out what was "normal" for each developmental stage. When they were scared of clowns or they told a white lie, it was reassuring to know that certain behaviors are common at certain ages. My mom was a resource in the baby years, but school kids and teens are in such a different atmosphere than Mom's day, you need some additional help. Reading *The Essential 55* together would be a preemptive strike for elementary and middle school kids, outlining success tips for school like "say thank you within three seconds of receiving something" and "make eye contact when in conversation." Teacher/author Ron Clark finds that children learn better when they've got some basic behavioral lessons down, and this book could be added to the bedtime story in short bites. Even in the "golden years" from ages 7 to 11, you need books like Divinyi's *Good Kids, Difficult Behavior* for another point of view on strategies to use with defiant behavior. Counselor Joyce Divinyi spells out effective approaches that are 'win-win' for parents, teachers, and children.

Let teens and young adults own their own problems & solutions. Even in our self-esteem culture, winning isn't everything. Winning builds confidence; failing and trying again builds character. **Keep trying to get through to your child no matter what**, and you set that example. The teen culture that says it's cool to be hard, there are no rules, and everything can be trashed is really hard to live with, if you're a dreamy optimist like me. The kids have a saying," Save your drama for your Mama." Sometimes you just want to hide from the hysterics and avoid the irritation and confrontation, but you must stick up for what you believe as a parent. If you're divorced, you have to drag your ex along, too. But **the opposite of caring is not conflict; it's indifference**. It's your job to set limits and enforce them. When family members don't care, they don't argue. They say, "I'm fed up, I just can't put up with their stuff." And that's when you see the family that's no longer in touch; they no longer get together for holidays and special occasions.

To find help in setting boundaries and saying no, invite the parents of your children's' friends over for brunch or pizza, work at a school function, or just call and introduce yourself, so you can be in touch with each other when there's a question about something. It's helpful to hear how different parents handle things. Co-ed sleepover parties after a dance or prom are popular in our area, but it was new to me, so I called a few parents to find out what the deal is.

Your sister or another mom with older kids can be a guide to things like prom etiquette and teen parties—she's been there before and she knows what questions to ask. **Check the fruit on the tree before you take advice from someone.** For example, my buddy Myra, with three awesome young adults, can be trusted to have the optimum scoop on everything from college prep to appropriate gifts. Whatever you do, **get some information, don't try to run your life in a vacuum, but trust your gut.**

This is a world where 30% of ninth-graders have had intercourse. It's also a world where the Internet is central to teen lifestyles. Keeping the household computer in plain view is a good watchful step, but now there's a better one—snooping software. Unlike internet filters that block cheesy web sites, secretly installed programs like Child Safe, Watch Right and eBlaster provide "snapshots" of sites, chat rooms, and instant message sessions your child has been to and e-mails them to your computer at work. A difficulty here might be that your employer is probably already using this software on YOU, so a private second address might be optimal. Viewed as an "early warning system," this information could guide you in important conversations with your child. Those real-life talks help update the most important filter there is—the one between their ears. Not comfortable with snooping? That's fine, but you must then be comfortable with the consequences.

Accept that no matter what you say, don't say, or do, your teen may appear to be allergic to you. In high school, your teen may even be "spoiling the nest" on purpose, to make it emotionally easier to leave. At a time in your life when *you* often wonder if you're "losing it," your teen will be glad to assure you that, yeah, you are. Be affectionate and open even if your efforts are not acknowledged, but **set clear expectations of their behavior, its consequences, and how *you* want to be treated.**

Parenting Teens With Love and Logic is a great resource for all kinds of situations. Knowing that kids face all kinds of life-and-death situations long before they're on their own, authors Cline and Fay show you how to give your teen opportunities to be responsible and allow them to live with the natural consequences of their mistakes. Avoid anger, threats, and power struggles using the "parenting pearls" in the end of the book, on topics such as backtalk, peer pressure, the silent treatment (you thought your kid was the only one?), and curfews. Calmness and respect wins, anger and lecturing lose. "Grandma will be disappointed if you don't come" beats "Because I said so!"

Anticipate tricky situations by asking questions like "What would you do if Heather met some guys and asked you to go with her in their car?" A safe place to bring this stuff up is riding in the car, and shopping trips are great places to find out what's going on in their heads. Between the ages of 17 and 21, there *will* be drinking going on at their parties. I think it's better to 'fess up to it, instead of tip-toeing around and everybody pretending it's not happening.

Discuss who's going to be the designated driver on the way home, and make it clear that your child can duck into the bathroom, call you on the cell phone if things aren't going well, and you'll come and park around the corner for a cool, minimal-explanation pick-up. Remember how the discomfort of your ninth month of pregnancy made you ready to give birth? The teen years make you ready to give birth to a college student or working adult! God definitely has a plan!

Being a mother is a tough job, but being a stepmother is even tougher! Step moms who've been on the battle lines say you've got to be involved – those kids are not going away, and neither are you. Have fun and hope they join in, and don't worry about sloppiness, mild rudeness, or sadness; they're kids and stuff will improve as they grow if you're patient, polite, and positive. Don't criticize the ex-wife and never, ever compare anything about your kids and your step kids. Step dad always needs to know when he can look forward to time alone with you, and at some point you should initiate "the conversation" about when and how everyone will be launched and out of the house. Regarding the step kid who just won't let you in—many of these tough nuts later say, "I didn't care for her/him, but I appreciated the way she/he was there for my parent." Not awesome, but better than banging your head against the wall.

The off-to-college phase is another new minefield, and the definitive guide, in it's third edition, is *Letting Go: A Parent's Guide to Understanding the College Years*. Authors Karen Coburn and Madge Treeger, a college administrator and a counselor, tell you how college life has changed and continues to evolve. In the three years between my first child's applications and my second's, the normal date for getting applications in changed from February to October and the foreign language requirement went from optional to imperative! Coburn and Treeger bring you up to date, starting you in the junior year of high school and taking you expertly through the orientation and freshman process. Their take on the mind-set of today's college students can help you open up a dialogue with your young adult.

The dad who hasn't shared in the dialogue in high school may jump in during college on e-mail. He may be more comfortable "choosing his words" in writing than engaging in spontaneous personal or phone chat. When your student gets acclimated to her new life, usually around February of freshman year, you may be surprised by a great leap in maturity. Guys, in particular, start taking better care of themselves and their possessions and complaining when roommates and project partners don't pull their weight. Resist the urge to comment on *their* recent stupidities, and just be glad you got to this place.

In *Letting Go*, impressions from other parents let you know that you're not the only one feeling disoriented after the big drop-off. The day you drop off your youngest is kind of a Wizard of Oz experience—one day you're in Kansas and outside forces are telling you what to do; the next day you're in Oz and *you* have to make all the new choices.

I don't believe you can totally wing it or gut it out over these years. Knowledge is definitely power and attitude is everything in this most precious area of your life. The pace of life is so fast right now, situations can deteriorate to Dad and Son in a defiance match or Daughter moving in with her boyfriend before you know it. Keep talking, talking, talking—with a professional in the middle, if need be—so that love and not one-upmanship is guiding family life. Share these books with Dad or talk him through what you've read so you can both be on the same page in responding to crises. Don't let things get to the point where there's a standoff and the family disintegrates. **Remind each other how you swore you'd never act like your parents! The only way to be different is to learn from the experts or from successful parents who are further down the road.**

The Checklist

❏ I. Dads, tell your daughters they're beautiful, strong, and smart. My father's comments still resonate in my soul.

❏ 2. Ask PTA leaders to list PTA meetings and committee opportunities in the fall for the entire year so you can work them into your calendar. Flyers posted at local supermarkets and drugstores help to remind working parents. Scheduling a PTA event on the same day as parent-teacher conferences makes time sense.

❏ 3. Don't fight it—restructure family vacation plans if bringing friends along is important to them. They have more fun and they're often better behaved, because they don't like to get yelled at in front of their friend. This is a great time to bring a same-age cousin along and strengthen family bonds. Whether friend or kin, explain to your kids that you need to share *your* vacation with someone you can trust and feel comfortable with.

❏ 4. Fight to sit down for meals together as often as possible. Research points to this as a big predictor for success in school. A "family night" needs to be flexible with athletic, rehearsal, and social commitments. Why not a "family Sunday lunch"?

❏ 5. The concept that oral sex is less intimate than intercourse is widely held among teens and young adults. Even one of our presidents thought so, so it's up to you to dispute it. I like "Dr. Phil" McGraw's definition—if it involves two people and their genitals, it's sex. This is one of those third person, car-ride talks.

❏ 6. Support for abortion rights has been dropping due to the decline in teen pregnancies, acceptance of single parenthood, and focus- shift from woman's rights to the rights of the fetus. Don't equate youth with liberal opinions; many teens are against abortion.

❏ **7.** Don't feel you can't discourage marijuana use because you tried it in your younger days. Today's weed is much stronger and is often laced with other chemicals. A recent Australian study found that teens using pot were twice as likely to experiment with or become dependent on drugs and alcohol. Didn't yo' mama say that?

The Checkup from the Neck Up

❏ My children are growing into their true selves, and I can't wait to meet the people they will become.

❏ I'm not in a hurry to rush to the next thing; I'm truly present in the moments of my kids' growing up, soaking up the sights, sounds, and smells of our lives together.

❏ My eyes light up each time I see my children. Though they may back away at times, I stay close, let them know they matter, and that they have everything it takes to have a great life.

10.

Empty Nesters and Boomerang Kids

Just when you get used to the empty nest, they're baaa-aack!

"Suddenly it seemed strangely familiar—as if I'd been on that innertube, sliding down that hill, hurtling through space for a very long time. Much like the last year of my life, when I'd seen time and again just how little control I had over my life, let alone the lives of those I loved. Couldn't stop my husband's illness. Couldn't prevent my mother's death. Couldn't keep my children from growing up. It's hard work, tedious and exhausting—isn't it?—trying to control the uncontrollable. What I felt on that hill was not fear, but fatigue. I was bone tired. So I simply let go. It was not easy to do, but I did it. Just opened my eyes, felt the wind in my hair, leaned back and enjoyed the ride. My husband was impressed. I'd forgotten how good it feels to live with abandon —to live in the present without fearing the future, without longing for the past. I won't forget it soon."
—**Sharon Randall**, in the ultimate mother-love book,
<u>Birdbaths and Paper Cranes</u>

My youngest left for college on August 31. I left two wall calendars open to August several days into October, as if August was the month the world ended. When I ask other new empty-nester parents how they're doing, there's a silence or a long "uhhhhhh," followed by "It's awfully quiet around here." The unspoken phrases are, "This is harder than I thought it was going to be," and "I have to find some way to fill up my time" and "I wish I hadn't yelled about messy rooms, cause now they're empty." (Not to mention the emptiness of your bank account, but more on that in Chapter 23)

My response has been to expand into my children's spaces. I love to nap in their beds and look at the pictures on their bulletin boards and the plastic stars on their ceilings that glow in the dark. I wear their old sweatshirts, marked Beverly Hills 90210 or Soccer All-Stars. I moved into their bathroom, my Time Defiance skin cream taking the place of their pore-destroying cleansing pads. I imagine widows do this when their husbands are gone, closing the door to the closet and holding the sleeves to their faces, drinking in the traces of cologne and shoe polish. I can still smell White Shoulders on my mother's ring and her pearls, sent to me in a manila envelope by the nursing home when she died seven years ago.

What am I doing here? Trying to recapture those crazy days of yesteryear, when you never knew what forgotten team practice or unresearched term paper would pop up? Trying to pretend everything was rosy, to deny that I often felt like I should get the Bad Mother Award? No, just remembering, grieving a little, and filling the empty spaces. I am learning to live in today and tomorrow in a new way. My consciousness is expanding and my knowledge of my own strengths and the potential of my future is growing daily. I'm becoming fiercely positive and lovingly tough; wise like Devorah and tough like

Esther, involved in a Rocky-style training period for the rest of my life. At some point my new life will be so gigantic, I may not *fit* into my old life.

When your kids are away, some positive things should be happening in your life. You and your mate may have more time to be sexual with each other, you can step up your spiritual studies and exercise program, and you can ramp up your professional life with a part-time business, graduate school, or training in new skills. I've enjoyed reconnecting with girlfriends via e-mail, telephone, and hanging out. Privacy, order, and a calm atmosphere may seem weird at first, but you'll actually get to like it. Mornings and evenings are relatively crisis-free, and there are just fewer times when you absolutely have to do something or be somewhere. The empty nest has become the quiet, convenient nest.

Many women choose to go back to school, starting or finishing those degrees they always meant to get. When your employer will pay, it's especially enticing to hit the books and ruin the curve for all those young people who aren't as sure they want to be there as you are. My friend Audrey is finishing the degree she started 20 years ago at Columbia, before her first son was born. She gets smarter than her usual extremely smart self every day! Carol's school system will be footing the bill for her masters in education degree, raising her salary to a level that will be reflected later in her retirement pay. Myra's getting her second master's degree, this time in public administration, opening the door to leadership in school or government agency settings.

Still, you may see a young mother on the street corner with a toddler and an infant, and wish to share their sweet wonder and feel those chubby arms around you again. I miss the certainty of knowing every extra minute of the day was already spoken for and every effort was intrinsically worthwhile. I miss the nookie you only get from carrying kids in your arms and their hugs and kisses. I miss Halloween costumes, apple-picking, and birthday parties. (My friend Claudia calls this "grandmother envy.") At work, you can't use the family excuse anymore; you may have to either fully engage or move on. If you were home for a while, you have to make a list and decide what to do with your time, taking responsibility for each day's success or failure instead of going with the flow of family life. Now you have new options, you have to make decisions, go forward, fail, succeed and once again set a new kind of example for those young adults wondering what Mom is up to.

Dad may be having an especially hard time. No matter whether he views his working life as successful or not, he may still grieve for the career road he *didn't* take or the family time he *should* have taken. In an effort to cover his confusion, he may talk about having another child or lash out at you; try to find the meaning behind the words. In the first episode of The Soprano's, 40ish Tony Soprano has been caring for and enjoying a family of geese living in his swimming pool. They fly away, of course, and Tony's grief is so intense he seeks help from a therapist to sort it all out. The sweet, simple geese were so much easier to understand than a complicated teenager, cantankerous mother, and midlife wife. My friend Aaron was greeted every day after work by a stray cat who hung out on his front porch. "Mr. Kitty" had become part of the family, until he came down with feline leukemia and had to be put down. It could be felt as another loss, on top of the loss of the last child moving in to her own apartment.

The empty nest may appear at first to be a loss. As I progressed through my youngest child's senior year of high school, I wondered what would replace the soccer matches, band concerts and plays when he left for college. Each family vacation seemed increasingly precious, knowing how difficult it is to steal time from busy calendars. Those bright spots on my calendar must be replaced with work, service and entertainment that I create for myself. The well-worn, happy path of parenthood has come to a fork, and we have to be alert to new opportunities to reach out to life.

Boomerang Kids Meet Boomers

> *"Human beings are the only creatures on Earth*
> *that allow children to come back home."*
> —Bill Cosby

But don't get too blissed out in your nest. When college is over and the new job hasn't kicked in with rent money yet, it may be time for the kids to boomerang home for a while. According to the Census, 18 million adults ages 18-34 live with their parents, up 42% since 1970. They're not slackers – the realities of the job and housing markets are tough today. Among 20-somethings, returning to the family nest has become not just acceptable, but expected, if you're pursuing an arts-related dream, trying to find yourself, or just can't find an appropriate job.

The first order of business, then, is to define "for a while" and to have a plan for independent living for all. Make a list of current expenses: car payment, insurance, and maintenance; health insurance; food, clothing, and entertainment; and phone/cell phone fees. Add a security deposit and probable monthly rent and utilities to that, and you have the figures your young person needs to shoot for. Then come up with a plan to reach this income goal, whether through a full-time job, new business, or multiple part-time commitments. Put a date on it, because a dream becomes a real goal when there's a date on it. Only when all these figures are on paper can he really know the price of independence. Even my right-thinking daughter kept mentally figuring only rent as her goal, until this total list brought the actual cost of supporting herself into sharper focus.

A scary fact of life in the 2000's is that there may be times—especially when your kids are in their 20's—when they're not covered by health insurance. Either they're looking for a job or they're training for a different one, but the bottom line is that most family health coverage ends when the kid graduates from college, when they turn 20-something, or both. I started telling other parents of college students about this at a holiday party, and some of them looked like they were going to be sick. They'd never thought about it, and the collective feeling was, "Does the financial obligation never end?!"

You certainly don't want this one to back up on you and destroy your entire financial picture. What are you going to say when your young adult needs medical attention? "Sorry, I can't afford it?" You need to take care of this one regardless of other demands. For example, health insurance is more important than having an apartment or making a car payment. Moving home and mooching a ride to school will have to fall into line with that $100-$400/month insurance payment. Welcome to real life, young person.

When your adult child moves in, draw up a 'contract' with expectations about percentage of time socializing versus job-searching and/or working, laundry, meals and chores, and have everyone sign it. Supply youth-oriented books like *10 Insider Secrets to Job Hunting Success!* by Todd Bermont, articles about effective interviewing and career searches, and interactive career quizzes like the one on focuscareer.com. Contact your doctors, dentists, neighbors, and friends to see if they know executives who'll hire new graduates, and encourage your kid to work for peanuts to learn new skills.

Remind your kids how annoying their sloppy, thoughtless roommates were, so they'll resolve not to be like them in their new role at home. Scott and I wouldn't be comfortable with having a boyfriend or girlfriend sleep over in the same room, and we've made that clear. We stay in touch via cell phone when we're on the road, and we expect our young adults to do the same. If you're going to stay overnight at a friend's house or stay out late, fine—just let someone know. That's what adults do. You may provide basics needed to get around, but fancy cars and feature-laden cell phones are something they buy when they have a full-time job and live on their own. Education expenses are a "family debt" to be paid off by any kid who makes it big. Some parents may ask for rent, and that can foster a sense of responsibility. Whether you use the money for expenses, to pay off a school loan, or save for their wedding or house purchase, that's up to you.

It's critical that the whole family discuss that you don't know how long you'll be able to perform and produce income to finance the long life you're expecting. It's vitally important during midlife to sock some money away for those sunny and rainy days only God knows about, and the sooner you start the easier it will be. This seems so obvious, but your child may not have thought about the fact that you need to do this now. Even if you have scads of money and you can afford to support your young adult in grand style, did it ever occur to you that you're doing them a disservice?

Remember the caterpillar-to-butterfly experiment you did in middle school? You watched as the caterpillar labored over its cocoon and the new butterfly struggled to emerge from its cocoon. That struggle helped to shape the butterfly's wings for flight. Maybe a student clipped an edge off the cocoon, making it easier for the butterfly to emerge, but that creature's wings were never right because it didn't go through the natural struggle of change. Humans are the same way. You have to let them struggle and learn to fly!

The fact is that Midlife Mamas and their children often have a lot more in common than we had with our parents. Sexuality, race, and women's rights were issues that polarized boomers and their parents, but the gap between boomers and their children is much smaller. Two recent AARP studies showed that people aged 18 to 57 were similar when it came to "levels of satisfaction, hopes for the future, and general world views." I've lived a similar life to my children's, so I can more easily relate to their issues than my parents, who were high-school educated children from large immigrant families.

Perhaps we can look forward to a mother-son conversation like this one, from *The Saving Graces*, by Patricia Gaffney: "He asked me if I liked being a stay-at-home mom. I looked at him curiously…'Yes, I liked it,' I said. 'Usually. Did you think it old-fashioned of me not to have a job?' 'No,' he said, sounding surprised. 'Anyway, you were always doing something. It's not like you were eating bonbons and watching the soaps. You made the home,' he said seriously. 'You were the home maker'…This was a new kind of conversation we were having. It happens to most of us eventually, the moment when our parents become real people, with motives and hopes as authentic as our own…"

P.S. The same conversation could be had with a working mom—"You were a role model and taught me to be a better, more self-reliant person." Have you had a positive conversation like this with *your* parent, admiring actions you observed growing up? It would mean so much to them!

There will have to be boundaries in any adult relationship, keeping private things private and yet being open to intimacy without being stepped on. Your kids don't "owe" you anything except respect and decent interaction; you don't "allow" them things you wouldn't "allow" any other adult. Watch for those words in your interactions, along with "you should've known." Everyone will make mistakes and trip over boundaries, but the main thing is that you both keep trying. The saddest thing I've seen is when adult children and their parents are indifferent and totally divorced from each other. I think we'll find that moving from a caretaking relationship to a friendship and teamwork role is easier than it was for our parents, as long as lots of listening and respect get thrown into the mix. There will be new boundaries, but sharing life with the people I love best in the world can only be a great thing!

The Checklist

❏ **I.** COBRA is a 1986 law that mandates up to 3 years insurance coverage for young adults who outgrow their parents' plans. It's expensive ($150-400), but good coverage, vital for preexisting conditions. Check with your benefits office as graduation approaches. Short-term policies for a couple of months can be purchased online at goldenrule.com or fortishealth.com. An individual $100/month Blue Cross-type policy with a high deductible will cover a catastrophic problem, but leave you holding the bag for checkups and routine care.

❏ **2.** After college is prime time for grandparents to do some tax-free gifting. At this point, the money can be used to pay off school loans without affecting scholarship eligibility.

❏ **3.** When it's time to plan the wedding, get *Bridal Bargains: Secrets to Throwing a Fantastic Wedding on a Realistic Budget.* Listen closely for what the kids want, welcome your new family members, and walk softly if you're the mother of the groom.

❏ **4.** Aging boomers bunking up with the over-70 crowd? After a midlife divorce or a senior's devastating illness, midlifers and seniors can buy more flexibility and peace of mind by moving in together and sharing expenses, child and invalid care, and hopefully, lots of laughs and loving gestures. *All Grown Up: Living Happily Ever After With Your Adult Children* by sociologist Roberta Meisel, asks longevity revolution questions like "What will your children need from you when they're 40 and 50 years old?" You'll still have a special power in your relationship even then, so will you be able to listen without interrupting?

The Checkup from the Neck Up

❏ I'm a good tongue-biter and offer advice only when it's appropriate. I listen carefully to my adult children, and seldom ask when they plan to: a)lose weight b)get a better job c)get married d)start their family e)save money.

❏ I celebrate the differences between me, my husband, and my children and their friends and "significant others." I choose to be the glue that holds my family together.

❏ I make time for my family and gladly choose to give of myself and my time to set the example for their futures. I balance this with taking good care of myself, so I can truly enjoy my family.

11.

Last Chance Midlife Mommies

Hey—I'm 40 and I forgot to have kids!

Help wanted ad for parents—Team Player with excellent communication and organization skills to work frequent 24-hour shifts. Must commit for life to a high quality product without complaining or expecting to be appreciated. No financial compensation—you pay them and a huge exit bonus at age 18 may or may not guarantee financial independence. Benefits include lots of laughs, hugs, and unlimited opportunities for personal growth.

Many positive, successful people celebrate a late 40's birthday and suddenly realize they won't be able to start a family. They produced so much work and wealth, they forgot to reproduce. They were so busy, it always seemed too soon to bring a baby into the picture. Now, it's too late. Some never met the right partner, and didn't want to start the process without one. Some were having such a good time, and they didn't hang out with people who had children, so it didn't occur to them. Some arrived at the end of a long series of fertility procedures empty-handed, ready to punch out on the biological clock. Some wish they had made a conscious decision about the issue, instead of letting the years make it for them. Denial, anger, confusion, feeling as if an important choice has been taken away – all the stages of grief have to be gone through, just as if you had lost a loved one.

Adoption—a blind date for life!

But it's not too late—there are children all over the world languishing in orphanages, yearning for a family. And lots of people your age are doing it—just type "international adoption" or "adopting older children" into your search engine and read the amazing stories of people just like you who are making it happen.

With one from Korea and one from Peru, my friends Rick and Libby are the poster family for international adoption. They're the first to admit that you'd better be a good team with some true grit to get this job done in your 50's, but they wonder what they did with their time before kids, like all parents. A good place to start learning about international adoption is the National Adoption Information Clearing House at *www.calib.com/naic*. Children from America are the focus of Downey Side America. Go to Kidsave.com to find out about a program called Summer Miracles that brings kids from Russia and Eastern Europe over to summer camps and places them with families for "try-on" periods.

For the single woman who's been searching the horizon for Mr. Right-Father-of-my-Child, the day may come when there are three options: adoption, artificial insemination, or man of the moment. If the risk of future custody disputes is a concern, artificial insemination offers more control. It takes persistence, courage, and money and you can face a lot of resistance from your family, friends, co-workers, and your employer, but if it rings true with you and you're 42 or under, go for it!

Alice Domar's *Conquering Infertility and Dr. Richard Marr's Fertility Book* have the latest info for couples trying to get in under the wire. Have a can-do attitude, relax knowing that you have the option to adopt, but don't go on any business trips when the thermometer says it's ovulation time!

Why do I feel so strongly about midlife mommies?

1. Because having my children is the single best thing I've ever done, right up there with marrying Scott.

2. Because I'm adopted, and I thank God someone cared enough to love and raise me.

3. Because you have 30 or 40 more years to reach for the stars, and it'll be fun to bring along some starlets and moonbeams!

12.

Husbands & Wives, Best Friends to the End

"By requiring more from yourself and your partner, you are, in essence,'changing the deal.' And make no mistake: Those with whom you are currently in relationships won't like it. They will resist your changing the status quo. You taught them the rules, you've been rewarding their conduct, and they, like you, have gotten comfortable with the deal. If the price of poker is about to go up, it's only fair that you warn them about the changes before you begin to respond to their behavior in a different way."
—**Phillip C. McGraw, Ph.D.**, Life Strategies

Back in 1992, John Gray's Men are from Mars, Women are from Venus helped men and women understand their differences by seeing ourselves as two species who have come to share the same planet and use the same language, but *understand* that language differently. At midlife, some of the old barriers come down, but have you given up yet on trying to make your husband just like you? That's like trying to make a pig fly!

Let's review, just in case you're still waiting for that pig to fly—women give unconditional love and men keep score;

women offer help without being asked and men think that's rude; women want to feel understood and cared for and men want to be respected and appreciated; women argue for the right to be upset and men argue for the right to be free; women want to share their feelings and men can't listen without trying to fix feelings; women want to talk about problems, while men want to go into their caves to solve problems so they won't be seen as incompetent; women give too much when they fear they're unworthy, while men stop giving when they fear failing or being seen as incompetent. These characteristics are not cast in stone, they're just tendencies to be dealt with. They apply to your teenage son as well as your husband. The take-home message for me has been—**your man will be most comfortable with a moderate amount of giving and communicating (too much makes him uncomfortable) and a maximum amount of compliments, respect, and admiration from you.**

Gary Chapman's concept of *The Five Love Languages* clarifies and "de-genders" the idea that Mars and Venus are speaking foreign languages to each other. Chapman shows that you primarily speak one of five love languages: "Words of Affirmation, Quality Time, Receiving Gifts, Acts of Service, or Physical Touch." One of these is the thing that makes you feel most loved. For example, I feel loved when a person says they appreciate me and gives me verbal compliments and kind and encouraging words—Words of Affirmation. Scott would be inclined to say that talk is cheap and actions are what count – Acts of Service. He would agree with Golde in Fiddler on the Roof: "For 25 years I've washed your clothes, cooked your meals, cleaned your house, given you children, milked the cow. After 25 years, why talk about love right now?"

The problem comes when you try to communicate in *your* language instead of your partner's language. Scott tries to show love to me by working very hard and completing all kinds of tasks around the house. I compliment him and express appreciation for what he does. **But we should both be doing the opposite.** I need to put anything he needs me to do first on my list, and think of *actions* that will make his life easier; that's speaking his language. He needs to take every opportunity to say kind, complimentary *words* to me, and guard against angry, harsh comments. Get it?

Think of your parents, siblings, children and friends—what makes their faces light up? Communicating *your* needs in *their* language and finding out what people *really* want doesn't come naturally; it's a choice that you make every day if you want to keep your relationships moving forward.

I've also kicked up the affectionate words, gestures, and touching since I read a survey that revealed **men rated lack of affection right behind a lack of sex as a cause of stress in their marriages.** *Affection?* You mean when you hug him and he immediately wants to jump on your bones? Yes, that will be his response if it's been a while, but if affection *and* sex are regularly on the menu, hugs will stop being a cue for The Act and just be reassuring. Anything that says "the fun and surprises just keep on coming" is good, along with any scalp massage, shoulder rub, or peck on the cheek that says "you are just so darn *cute.*" A "you turn me on" card for absolutely no reason, a tight full-body hug, and a butt grab are actions that mean as much as your intention to stop nagging. I realized recently that holding hands and having his arm around me in public turns me on, so I *asked* Scott to do it. He does, and I love it! *Any* tiny move toward reciprocating your affection should be rewarded with enthusiasm!

Another common mistake married folks make is "dubbing in"—deciding what your partner is thinking without asking.

You catch him staring at your butt and think "He can't believe how huge it is," when what he's really thinking is "I'd love to have sex tonight." He hasn't spoken to you all day, so you wonder what's bothering him, while he's thinking "it's nice and peaceful today."

Are there more fights than good times in your marriage? Are they about **who has control and who gets to be right?** You be the one to stop the argument from escalating and say "Let me just listen to what you're saying for a minute." Drop the name-calling, "you said/I said," "You never" and "You always." Lower your voice and say things like "Can I please just tell you what I was thinking?" "What are we fighting about?" and "I hate to fight." Do you want to be right or do you want to be happy? If someone has to win, then someone has to lose.

Is there a male menopause?

Yes, there are some physical changes related to hormones in men over 40: 52% experience some form of erectile dysfunction; emotional symptoms include irritability, indecisiveness, and depression; and sleep, memory, and weight problems are common. Sound familiar? Problems arise when your man thinks *you're* the problem and/or that he's the only guy with these changes. Guys don't "share" this stuff; they've spent their whole lives exaggerating how much weight they can lift, how much money they're making, how big the fish was, how big their penis is, how many orgasms they've had, and how many sexual partners they've had. It's highly unlucky he'll ask the guys at work if they're feeling restless and unfulfilled. And when he sees *you* struggling with your weight, your periods, and those sprongy grey hairs, it breaks through his expert denial to remind him that *he's* getting older too.

You are now in the "midlife crisis" zone. Hopefully he won't head for the two extremes of this zone—completely blowing up his current life or feeling powerless and becoming completely depressed. Maybe he really believes for a few moments that 20-something Courtney in accounting wants *him*, not his job; or maybe he gets depressed when that really-fit-guy-his-age at the health club takes the Stairmaster to heaven and drops dead. He may struggle with the idea that life doesn't go exactly as planned, and no amount of oat bran, vitamins, and extra push-ups can fix that.

Sometimes a man has to reflect on the worthiness of youthful dreams. Others have reached the Promised Land and found that the milk is sour and there's no honey, that professional success hasn't delivered a neat package of happiness. Some goal adjustment is called for; don't try to prop up the corpse of old dreams and do the Don Quixote. Sit shivah and grieve for the old goals, set some new ones, and take up a sport that gets both of you out in the sun. No, the convertible, the hair transplant, and the liposuction probably won't help; he'll just be "the older guy with the plugs and the hot car." We're not talking cynicism, despair, and surrender here, just writing a new mission statement for the second half of life!

Talking to a live, feisty counselor at his level is, of course, the optimal goal, though I'm not sure how well Tony Soprano is progressing through *his* therapy. Maybe a little "cinema therapy" would help get your man on the road to taking a hard look at the rest of his life. Start with three midlife comedies — *Groundhog Day*, *Down and Out in Beverly Hills*, and *Defending Your Life*—that are hysterical treatments of the man-meets-midlife theme. If he can laugh at this transition, then he can move on to books like Harold Kushner's *When All You've Ever Wanted Isn't Enough* and *Living a Life that Matters*, using the biblical lessons of Ecclesiastes and Jacob in a very relatable way to explain the tough questions. In Howell Raines' *Fly Fishing Through the Midlife Crisis*, the folksy author progresses from The Redneck Way (conquering the fish) to a more relaxed, throw-the-fish-back style of life. For guys who don't like to read, these are available on tape and CD. The main point of it all is for your partner to know that midlife is a well-worn path we all walk, and that the uncomfortable feelings will tell us some things, if we'll only listen.

Imagine if they engraved your outstanding characteristics on your gravestone! Some women's stones would read "Always there for the family, fantastic cook, clean refrigerator." Mine would say "Always knew where the party was!" Scott never has to fear that we'll have nothing to do on the weekend; I've usually got it booked up months in advance. Yet, many couples get in a rut with this stuff, always seeing the same old people and doing the same old things. Magical, spontaneous moments require advance planning, especially for couples in a groove so deep, it's a rut. Recent studies have shown that having new adventures together freshens every area of a relationship.

Try spending Saturday doing what he wants and Sunday doing what you want. Take a Karate, dance, or investment class together, sleep naked for a change, or take a seasonal part-time job together to save up for a cruise. **Be as polite to each other as you are to strangers**, and point out little things he can do for you while you step and fetch for him. Get away from the familiar drone of the TV, the comfort of the couch, and the illusion that you're "getting things done." Recall the days when your courtship was fresh and you were trying to impress each other with your hunger for life. A friend of mine never found out her husband wanted to tour local art museums—until they had separated and he was filling the kids in on his activities with his new girlfriend!

When your He-Man Klingon gets clingy…

Most men form no new friendships after the age of 30. Just when you're spreading your wings and piling up new friends, your husband seems to be clinging to you in a whole new way. You can help maintain connections with school buddies, friends from work, and brothers—and develop that new acquaintance with the assistant soccer coach—by making the extra effort to invite them to summer barbecues and setting up an occasional dinner-out-date. Try to overcome any problems with the friend's wife, a seemingly inevitable complication of couple relationships that can cause you to hesitate when you pick up the phone.

My friend Jack formed a group of 60-plus men who have a monthly dinner date. They call themselves the ROMEO's— Real Old Men Eating Out. If your man is ready to kick it up a notch, I'd encourage those wild-at-heart man get-togethers, like going fishing, boating, and camping; some kind of a road trip; attending a sports event; building something real, like a deck, or unreal, like battle-bots; or training for a race or contest together. Men need those get-togethers just like you need your girlfriend time, and let's face it—an exciting aspect of your man is that he is *not* exactly like you.

Why is *this* your responsibility *too*, you ask? You're right, it's not, but keeping your social horizons wide open like this keeps you flexible, and it's a loving thing to do for a socially-impaired mate. Let's face it—as the years go by, there are fights and even deaths that break up old relationships. You can become best friends with a woman you just met in the ladies room; most men can't do that. What was that your grandma used to say? "Make new friends, but keep the old; one is silver and the other's gold." Avoid the social isolation and dependence on you that becomes so noticeable at midlife by helping your husband with a little calendar planning.

Have you had "The Conversation" yet?

That's the one where you talk about how you want to spend the rest of your lives together. How much of the college expenses and weddings will we pay for the kids, and how will we do it? (Then let *them* know what the deal is when it's appropriate.) What do we picture ourselves doing from 50 to 60, 60 to 70, and beyond—working, helping out at the soup kitchen, playing golf, traveling, creating art, and pitching in with the grandkids? Where will we live?

You might bring this up during a car trip, preceding it with "One of these days, we have to talk about…," so he can think about it without feeling cornered. Don't be the couple who goes to the financial planner and finds to your mutual surprise that he wants to live in a cabin in the woods and you want to travel the world! Have at least a sketchy plan for the next 5, 10, and 20 years, so that all the little decisions along the way correspond with the plan.

Do I dress like Cher or Queen Elizabeth?

Now, class, what about the physical stuff? We're all tired of hearing sex is purely physical for men and emotional for women; those lines blur during midlife anyway, as men seek more connection and women seek…well, that's in Chapter 14. A friend said to me recently, "When do I get to stop looking like his honey, doing all this maintenance on my grey hair and teetering around on those stupid high heels he likes? He makes comments when I try to change anything." You may not like my answer—if he's still noticing, I'd keep up the maintenance. He loves you for your real self, but he needs that visual stimulation to keep that part of him going. "Trashy" is only for home viewing, but "trendy" can be adapted so that your man knows you haven't caved in to age and given up on trying to please the eye.

If you only describe your hairstyle as "It's easy to keep it neat," maybe it's really your anger at your partner that's being controlled. If your underwear starts to look like his and you and your husband wear the same polo shirts, I'd worry. When you're as worn, lumpy, and comfy-looking as his recliner, you'll get treated like furniture. When all your footwear could be worn on a hike, I wouldn't be surprised if he takes one. Hey, I'm not saying this is fair, but it's really effective! Showing your neck by wearing your hair up or showing a little thigh through the slit in your skirt says, "Yeah, I'm still interested" loud and clear. I can't picture fastening my garter belt at 70, but who knows? The alternative is to "act your age," make yourself comfortable, and see what happens. My guess is, if you don't look like you're looking for a great life, no one will help you create one. Do *you* check out men who're sloppy, grossly overweight, and look like they just don't care? Are *you* attracted by men who are so "neat" and out-of-style, they look sterile, or do you sigh over the wild long-haired hunks on the covers of romance novels? I've got to believe that God made men and women different for good reasons and that criticizing those differences makes no sense.

Don't panic if you and your husband haven't attained perfection in your marriage; change is the norm for relationships. Though there is that couple that seems to inhabit the same sunbeam, most couples continuously work to develop real love after they realize that romantic love and power struggles can't carry the load. People grow and change, or they get stuck somewhere and the marriage is constantly in a state of coping, resolving, and reconnecting. Even that drinker or gambler who has fallen down the 12 Steps a few times may turn it around in midlife and become that man you always knew was there. **Many couples in their 60's look back to the years since 40 and say, "I'm glad I stuck it out. Divorce wouldn't have solved anything and now my life has a wholeness that's fantastic!"**

Do you have a detailed vision of what you'd really like your relationship to be like? Do you want to stop being the couple who lives to fight, the passive couple who've just given up, or the convenience couple who has no spark? Stop the silent suffering and imagine what life could really be like. At first, you'll just think about the things you'd like to eliminate: "I wish he'd stop yelling and being angry at the world," "I don't want to fight about money," "I wish he'd watch less sports and help with the kids and home projects," "If he doesn't take better care of himself, he'll be dead," "He needs to stop complaining and find another job." If you jump on every bad move he makes, you'll be *very* right and *very* lonely. If you use fears, needs, and other secrets he's revealed to you against him, you'll be talking to the back of his head for a long time. Stop the blaming, finger pointing, and accusing and put your energy where it can do some good.

Take your focus off your Don't Wants and flesh out your Wants: "He shows he loves me with his devotion to the family," "I enjoy our weekly date night and the little weekends away that we take together," "His new focus on staying fit and saving money for the future is a great example to our family," "He compliments me on my efforts to improve our home and my appearance" "He tells others how proud he is of my success at work." Do the things you'd like *him* to do *yourself*, especially under the category of finding things to admire about your spouse. Your man needs your admiration more than you need his—that's wired into the gender. When he overhears you telling someone (like your children) how important his work is and how well he does it, his ability to be open to you grows. When you tell him how proud you are of what he does for the family, his confidence and trust in you grows.

He may be a little suspicious at first of your happy, forgiving attitude. When you stop trying to control and compete, concentrating on pursuing your joyful self, it will seem weird at first to *his* controlling, competing self. But as you paint your joyful canvas, you're handing him the paints and brushes to do the same thing himself. When you stop being a people-pleaser, nagger, worrier, and controller, you're setting a close-up and personal example of how to write a new script and live a sensational life!

The Split that Hits Hard

Midlife divorce is so prevalent, it's a cliché, and yet each person going through it thinks they're the only person who feels trapped by the financial responsibilities and the kids; by the yearning to be admired again when your spouse takes you for granted; by the feeling that you've grown and your partner hasn't. A psychiatrist friend of mine who doesn't usually make generalizations told me that women leave a marriage just because it's not working for them emotionally; men will stay in a crummy marriage until they've found another partner. Women are often able to share their feelings with friends and find that others have found a way through this, while men seem to plan their escape or pursue their new partner in private without the perspectives gained from friendly viewpoints. The result is that men are often further down the road toward leaving when the relationship starts to unravel.

If you feel that your partner already has one foot out the door, or even if he has recently left, you can still attempt to save your marriage. Michelle Weiner Davis's *The Divorce*

Remedy contends that one committed partner can take specific action steps to bring the marriage back from the brink of divorce. Her proven track record addresses issues like infidelity, depression, Internet obsessions, sexual problems, and the famed "midlife crisis." **If you think it's just not 'fair' that one person has to start all the compromising and changing, you're right, but the stakes are so high, particularly if you have kids.** Their live-in dad is the guy most likely to love and care for them and older kids have a hard time "letting in" any new partner of yours emotionally. Besides, don't you want to be able to say "I did everything possible to save my marriage?" Second marriages have an even more dismal failure rate than originals at over 63%, but I pray you'll have the time of your life with your true soul-mate.

As a friend to a couple in trouble, the best thing you can do is to urge them to keep trying and I don't mean just going to counseling (though that's a must.) Yes, they have to learn new ways to respect each other, but don't *you* be the one who urges her to "throw the bum out" because he won't meet her half way. Someone usually has to purposefully start the changes, focusing on the positive and sliding thorny issues under the rug temporarily until things lighten up. Marriage has never been a 50/50 proposition; both must give 100%. Urge patience, compromise, and keep the emphasis on the long view of what your friends really want. **They should know that many people have felt as they do. "I feel trapped," "I'm just not in love anymore", "I feel dead inside", and "We haven't been good together in a while" are common refrains.** Just knowing that none of these is an original thought helps, and if you've personally worked through them, that's even more help to your embattled friend. Many are glad they hung around long enough to work on the relationship and rediscover what they loved about their partner.

Still, midlife is a time when many women choose to end an abusive marriage. The fantasy that your husband will change or the way you interact will change fades into the background, and someone either walks away, acts out through an affair, or decides to stay put in what may be called an emotional divorce. Maybe you're just tired and need to pursue some separate activities or maybe you are truly indifferent—that's the opposite of love. The only thing worse than being in a horrible relationship for 20 years is being in a horrible relationship for 20 years and one day!

The kind of abuse that *can* be most successfully renegotiated is verbal abuse, as described in two books by therapist Patricia Evans, *The Verbally Abusive Relationship and Controlling People*. **If your husband is a private anger addict and seems constantly irritated with you no matter what you say or do, that's verbal or emotional abuse.** You may doubt your feelings and feel confused since it won't happen in front of others, but you are not provoking it. He owns his anger, distancing, and disrespect, not you.

If there is name-calling like *idiot* or *bitch*, that's obvious. If you are trivialized, if many comments are countered, if there is a torrent of put-downs, cruel jokes, criticizing, and blaming, alternating with the cold shoulder and phrases like "You're too sensitive" and "I have no idea what you're talking about," you must read Evan's books. **This is not logical behavior that will go away if you "discuss" it; it comes from a family background of securing loved ones and feeling safe by belittling others.** You will be empowered to stop the mind games and calmly say " I dare you to repeat and think about what you just said. You will *not* talk to me like that." You will be helping, not hurting him. He doesn't want to be that way and he needs your help to change; if he doesn't, you can say you gave it your best shot. There are over 100 passionate customer reviews of Evans' books on Amazon.com, so I think it's safe to say that a lot of people are confronting this issue.

Yes, it could be boring to be with the same person for decades. So don't *be* the same person – keep changing, growing, and learning new things, staying fit, healthy and active. Encourage your partner to do the same. See yourselves together, in a life of continuous improvement.

The Checklist

❑ **I.** Guys enjoy "Dr. Phil" McGraw's bottom-line, humorous, man's-man style; even if your man wouldn't be caught dead reading a "marriage book," he'll see himself in McGraw's *Relationship Rescue*, on tape, CD, or in book form.

❑ **2.** For excellent advice if a divorce moves forward, own *Divorce and Money: How to Make the Best Financial Decisions During Divorce.* Author Violet P. Wodehouse is a family law attorney *and* financial planner, so you may know more than your attorney if you read it.

❑ **3.** For the scriptural, Christian viewpoint on saving your marriage, read *When Love Dies*, by Judy Bodmer.

❑ **4.** He should get the PSA test and keep the saw palmetto supplements around to chase away the prostate problems; 40% of men deal with it to some degree as they age. Nutrilite Saw Palmetto with Nettle Root is a sophisticated, cutting edge blend, and Schiff's Prostate Health uses the Excell form of selenium that's used in studies. For families dealing with it, some first-person accounts are *Hit Below the Belt and You Can't Make Love If You're Dead*.

The Checkup from the Neck Up

❏ I don't wait for my partner to change or "get it." I don't have to get his permission or cooperation to act lovingly. I have the power to control how I react to behaviors and situations. I create an atmosphere of harmony where communication can grow.

❏ I love offering a soft word of understanding, encouragement at a difficult time, a surprise gift, an affectionate gesture, a compliment, and lots of laughs.

❏ Whenever we disagree, I take the high road, stating specifically what I want. I avoid premature articulation, name-calling, and "You never/you always/you're nothing but a/ and you make me sick with your..." I forgive easily and give the first hug, the first goodnight kiss, and the first back rub.

❏ Being right is the booby prize of life. Insisting on being right makes my partner withdraw from me. When I recognize *all* the ways of being "right," I show generosity and goodwill and focus on friendship and what we enjoy about each other.

13.

Losing Your Virginity— the Second Time Around

"In a way both husband and wife are like Sleeping Beauty. Each would like the other to wake him or her from this sexually sleepy state. Maybe they harbor unspoken anger and hold private grudges. Maybe they are simply bored, with themselves and with each other. . .Are you waiting for your partner to rescue you sexually? Stop waiting. . .Light your own fire, and your partner will get caught up in the flames. You are about to become an irresistible sexual force."
—<u>Sex Over 50</u>, **Joel D. Block, Ph.D.**

Remember how you wondered about "the first time?" Would it hurt, would he know what to do, would you feel different after that? Maybe you had a wonderful experience, or maybe, like me, you were disappointed and wondered what all the fuss was about. All the romantic novels painted a rosy picture of your new relationship status, while you may have searched out magazine articles that detailed how to "get in the mood" when you really weren't.

If you were in your 20's, that was normal, because we now know that 20-somethings actually have the least sexual satisfaction of women of all ages, with uncertainty and dysfunction running at an all-time high. 30-somethings are often so busy with demanding careers and/or young families, they can't wait to get sex over with so they can get some sleep! After 40, you may still feel the pull to maximize career and family commitments, or you may feel bitter about your partner's lack of response to past efforts to change your sex life. Don't give up —you're just getting started, and the best is yet to come!

You laugh now when you think back to how you obsessed about "the first time," because sex may be a regular part of your life, whether it's twice a week or twice a month. If your husband spends years on his golf swing and minutes on sexual foreplay, enthusiasm may not be the word that comes to mind when you think about sex. Yet enthusiasm and wanting to be there is the #1 sexual characteristic valued by both men and women (*not* a sexy body, you cover-uppers).

We like to think that enthusiastic sex is perfectly natural, but that doesn't mean it's naturally perfect. Both of you have to acquire an attitude of continuous growth and change in your sex life, but one of you (probably *you*) has to get the ball rolling. Scott, in true manly style, crunched the numbers and figured out that we've probably made love over 3,000 times! Or, like a divorced friend of mine, you may be wondering if you can be reclassified as a virgin because it's been…a while. In either case, I'd like to propose that Midlife Mamas take a dramatic step and lose their virginity!

I'm proposing that you finally take responsibility for your own sexual satisfaction and growth. **When I say it's time for you to lose your virginity, I mean I want you to finally *do* all those things you've thought about doing over the years and *stop* repeating the following kinds of self-talk:**

- Real people/nice people don't do that.
- My man is a 'let's get to it' kind of guy.

- I'm afraid of looking foolish.
- What if the children hear/see?
- No one wants to have sex with someone who looks like me.
- I don't feel like it/ he doesn't feel like it.
- I'm too tired.
- I can't tell my partner what I need/ he never gets it.

Do you know what turns you on? Do you know *exactly* how to give yourself an orgasm? Some women have never bothered to find out where the bases are in the ballpark "down there." They've made love in the dark, in bed, with little conversation. In the bathtub or shower, or while taking a nap by yourself, let your hands and your biggest sexual organ (your brain) wander. Fantasize about someone you've seen or something you've read; get things tingly, but don't put pressure on yourself to have an orgasm unless you want to. Learn how to talk sex to yourself, focusing on your pleasure and not letting your mind wander. Have you thought about a bikini wax? He'll certainly go wild, but it feels so different, it'll get you in gear also. Practice privately and often, and then show your partner; it will both turn him on and educate him. Rhett Butler and the princes in fairy tales always knew what to do, but real men may not.

There are entire books on masturbation —learn some new tricks with *Tickle Your Fancy*, a book that takes self-pleasure to a new level, or learn from Betty Dodson, 71, the "grandmother of self-love," in her book *Sex for One*. The Berman sisters, the doctor/sex therapist team who authored *For Women Only*, may send women patients home with a prescribed, battery-operated device called Eros to "increase blood flow to the clitoris." British Female Inventor of the Year Liz Paul invented a clitoral stimulator called Vielle. It's a disposable device that fits over the finger, halves the time it takes for a woman to climax, and intensifies the orgasm. (Could be a whole new image for the name "Mrs. Paul".)

Five Minutes to Orgasm

Putting it all together is the book *Five Minutes to Orgasm Every Time You Make Love*, showing a simple technique to reach orgasm faster and more reliably during intercourse. Girlfriends, this is really not that mysterious. It's all about thinking sexy thoughts and the clitoris. Vaginal orgasm is a myth, except when vaginal thrusting *pulls* on the clitoris. You can do this without depending on the skills, timing, and foreplay of your partner, though all of that will improve too as you explore what turns *you* on. You and your lover can still light candles and spend hours making love; the *Five Minute* technique is for those quickie times when you just want to get it done.

Variation, choices, and not knowing what comes next are important to women during sex. Like a good mystery, sex is better for women when the details are new and different, revealed a little at a time. Our goal-oriented men, on the other had, like to follow a formula for success and go straight for it. Certain metaphors are apt; a woman is like an iron, a man is like a light switch; a woman is like a crock pot, a man is like a microwave. Women need time to heat up and find that doing things mechanically, instead of seeing where the sex will take you, is a turnoff. John Gray, as usual, has an interesting perspective in *Mars and Venus in the Bedroom*: "It is very important for a man to remember to go north before he goes south…Men should aim to have a feather touch down there. When the woman wants it harder, she can easily let him know by pushing her pelvis. . .While touching a woman's genitals, a man needs to remember to vary his approach. . .Sometimes it is good to grab a pillow and plan to camp out down south for a full fifteen minutes. You should just resign yourself to the fact that you are not going anywhere else for quite a while." If more men were this determined, there'd be a lot of happy woman out there!

Guide him with a sigh, moan, uh-huh, yes, mmm, and yeah; if you both like sexy talk, use it. Let your man know that doing different things makes you feel sexy: cuddling, massaging, wearing sexy clothes, watching a sexy movie, admiring yourselves in the mirror, acting out a fantasy, reading a passage from a sexy book, bathing and showering together. All these activities will keep you fresh and inspired for this and the next time.

Having better sex is a win-win goal in so many areas of your life. Your marriage and your health are obvious beneficiaries, and with the right attitude, you can add some daring sexual exploits to your "Life is Short" fun-and-adventure list. But did you ever think about sex as part of your spiritual journey? **I don't believe it's an accident that so many people say "Oh, God" when they come. We say "Oh, God" when something is intense, whether bad or good. Are we asking for help, praising, or feeling God's presence close at hand?** During orgasm, there is no thought, just feeling and connection with your partner and with…the divine? Many of us must need this release to be whole, in God's eyes and our own. We humans seek it with such intensity, it must be part of the plan pulling us closer to ultimate peace.

Speaking of seekers, check out the story of Jane Juska, author of *A Round-Heeled Woman: My Late-Life Adventures in Sex and Romance*. After 30 years of celibacy, this 66 year old, long-divorced, retired English teacher ran an ad with a box-number reply in the New York Review of Books personals. It read: " Before I turn 67—next March—I would like to have a lot of sex with a man I like. If you want to talk first, Trollope works for me."

Describing herself as "an easy sixty-seven year old lay," Juska's adventures with the men who answer her ad are not a geriatric fling, but a bittersweet stereotype-buster about older women with lingering libidos. When asked how she disrobed in front of strange men, she replied, "Quickly." Her well-written stories about teaching her love of great literature to high school students and prisoners make her yearning for a real love affair (she found one) more funny and real. I'm not saying what she did is a great idea, but if she's got the chutzpah to do *this*, you can definitely stir things up in *your* sex life!

Here's to you, Mrs. Robinson!

There's an urban legend out there that goes something like this: women get wild as they near menopause, and they pursue defenseless young men to satisfy their insatiable sex drives. Every guy has *heard* "from a reliable source" about these older woman ("You know, forty-five, fifty years old"), but you never actually speak to *the* guy who was attacked by one of these mad hormone-driven monsters. Tell me if you see one on *Jerry Springer* or *Jenny Jones*; tell me, just don't ask me to watch. These red hot menopause mamas are either the mother of a friend (like Mrs. Robinson or Stifler's Mom in the American Pie movies) someone at work, or a fellow traveler in a hotel, on a cruise, or at a resort. I'm not sure whether these legends are true or not, but where there's smoke, there may be women with hot flashes—who knows? It's intriguing to wonder—are they trying to get in under the wire with the hunk they never had? Are they really insatiable, or are their partners hiding, so they're striking out into new territory? Is the Change-of-Life lover proof of her newfound power, or some sort of anti-aging treatment for the hot-to-trot? We do know that the ratio of testosterone to estrogen increases at midlife, so the man-eating midlife mamma may not be just a myth.

That longing to get some great sex on her resume often coincides with a general determination to move ahead in all areas of life – and with an irritation at old roadblocks. "Look out world, here I come," is her motto. At the same time, her partner may be slowly losing testosterone or topped out in his profession, gotten laid off, or is generally feeling trapped. Health challenges feel like a punch in the gut. He may be puzzled by, or even resent, her new confidence.

The result may be that he suddenly has performance problems or withholds sex without even realizing the cause of all the confusion. It's the classic set-up for each to wonder if the other doesn't find them attractive any more. Remember, your man will do almost anything to avoid failure – like avoiding the situation altogether. The questions may seem too big to confront, and the cover-up begins. Nodding and smiling, the couple gives graduation parties and weddings, hanging onto the coat tails of their children's joy, all the while wondering where they left theirs. Those who started their families later become super-coach Dads and move-'em forward Moms, so wrapped up in their kid's lives, they don't have to examine their own. Take a lover, take a promotion— anything to avoid the pain.

Reveal to him how to romance you.

Recognize these scenarios for what they are—ways to avoid looking at what's really going on. Get a check-up and resolve any physical problems, and start *talking* to each other. If you ignore each other or argue for most of the day, don't expect the night to be filled with fantasy sex. Kindness, compliments, and shared laughter are the finest foreplay on the planet. The only way to reconnect is to cut through the anger, hurt, and indifference and start finding out

what you still love and admire about each other. Use the
teachable moments. When you ask him "How do I look?"
and he grunts, confess that what you're really looking for is a
compliment. " I was hoping you'd say I look pretty. That's
what I really want to hear. And I'd love it if you just
randomly said something like 'Hey, that's a great outfit' or
'You look terrific.'" Say what you want to happen, not in
anger, but in an open, hopeful way. If you want him to
come and hug you when you come home, make it easy for
him and tell him how much you appreciate it. If you want
him to end phone calls with "I love you," keep doing it
yourself. Establishing little romantic rituals help him be
successful in loving you.

If you've been rejected when you tried to initiate sex, it's
hard not to take it personally. If it happens repeatedly, back
off. Wear perfume, sexy underthings and nighties, or sleep
naked, letting him know you're in the mood. Try letting him
take the initiative, knowing that you're available. Give him a
chance to "fill in the blanks" and seduce you. If it's been a
while, try honestly stating what's bothering you—"I feel like
you don't want to have sex with me. Do you want to talk
about it?" If the answer is "Everything's fine," move on,
stop analyzing everything, and live a flaming life. It's probably
some situation at work he doesn't want to talk about.
Asking him to stroke you or massage you in bed may get him
back in the saddle.

There will be seasons when you're in sync, and some
when you're not, but whenever possible, *just do it.* He'll
flick on his light switch; you'll heat up your iron after 10
minutes of necking. He'll light up his microwave; you'll get
your crockpot heated up soon. It's a form of communication
that's worked well for humanity. It unifies a husband and

wife in a mystical way that surpasses shared experience, children, and property.

Take off your emotional clothes for each other.

You may have to start admiring him first outside the bedroom (uh-oh, here she goes again with that compliment stuff) to set the example, clear the air, and get things moving in the right direction. Tell him you were remembering how much he helped out when your mother was sick or how happy you are that he takes care of maintaining the cars and you don't have to think about it. Talk about sex when you're not tired or in bed, and focus on positive things you can do rather than "problems." When you both finally start talking, don't interrupt or contradict each other—feelings are feelings, they're not right or wrong. Create a trust zone, where feelings can be heard without being analyzed or judged. You don't have to answer everything; you can just say you heard and you're thinking about it. Bring up new sexual adventures ahead of time, giving both of you time to think about it. Establish when no is no.

Things won't suddenly get "solved," but over time you'll have little successes here and there. Don't be impatient – you are in the process of meeting in a whole new place, taking off your emotional clothes for each other. Remember back in the day when we used to call sex "fooling around"? Now it's like professional sports, with penalties for overtime. Let's relax, have fun, and start fooling around again. Go out on dates, leave the kids with Grandma for a weekend, have a sense of humor, and take responsibility for your sex life. He doesn't have to "give you" orgasms. You need to develop your own erotic lesson plan.

A Letter to Your Lover

Do women have a hard time talking about sex or do men have a hard time listening? There's probably a little bit of both in the mix, and the end result is the same—lack of communication leading to lack of sex. Feel free to photocopy this letter and put it on the seat of his car, in his lunch or briefcase, or in a card mailed to him, marked <u>confidential</u> —<u>not</u> under his pillow, to be read when he's tired. All these strategies allow him to think it over before he sees you, when he's clear about his feelings and opinions. Notice the results-oriented headline and the positive language, a good guide for how you should communicate in person. (It's also a great checklist of things you should do for him.)

I'd love to have more sex...

And I have a hard time telling you how much I enjoy
our love-making. For me, sex starts hours or days before
we make love, when you touch me as you pass by,
when you kiss me when you're going out, when you call me
or leave a message on my cell phone during the day,
when you thank me for something, tell me I look great
or I did something well. I feel turned on when you listen to me,
when you make plans for us to do something together,
and when you surprise me.

When I feel loved, I can't wait to make love!

Talking, listening,
being affectionate, helping with laundry and in the kitchen
so I have time for myself—this is what I call foreplay!
Rest, exercise, compliments, and knowing you want me—
    these are my aphrodisiacs!
When we're showered and smelling good, I love to make love
    slowly, with slow kisses, touches, and undressing. I feel like
    a goddess when we touch and caress each other everywhere!
And after these times, I can't wait 'till the next time!

14.

Sexual Fitness— Use It or Lose It

"You can fake blonde. You can fake tan. You can even fake sexy –
for a while. What you can't fake is the real and unmistakable scent
and feel of someone who actually likes sex. *You can't fake that*
Bessie Smith growl, the easy warmth of someone who wants a little
sugar in her bowl and who is prepared, under the right
circumstances, to have and give a very good time…The heart of
sexual energy is making others feel beautiful, wanted, clever,
charming. . .and appreciating what we have to offer as well as what
they, the lucky objects of our desire, do."
—**Amy Bloom**, in <u>O the Oprah Magazine</u>

Sometimes the spirit is willing, but you just can't lubricate.
Sometimes you just don't feel like it. Sometimes you feel like
it, but you don't have a partner. Sometimes, you have a
partner, but it takes you forever to orgasm. Sometimes you
have a partner, but he doesn't feel like it, he can't get started,
or he can't finish, because he's dealing with pressure at work,
diabetes, heart medications, or prostate enlargement. What's a
Midlife Mama to do?

The answer is simple: get a check-up, both of you, and find out if hormone changes, health problems, or medication are wrecking your sex life. Don't automatically attribute the fact that you don't "feel like it" to anger, aging, indifference, boredom or weight gain.

Find out why you don't have the response you used to. It's estimated that **70% of sexual problems over 40 are tied to treatable physical or emotional problems.** Get the proper medication, cut the booze, eat right, get some exercise, see the shrink, and slap a patch on your skin or a pill in your mouth. **Being a sexual woman in midlife will probably require more maintenance and investigation than it did at 30; deal with it.**

Fax or e-mail your doctor before the appointment to see if there's a problem with doing the tests in Chapters 26 and 21. Find out what your insurance will cover and pre-approve it. Go to bat for yourself, and you'll find the correct way to file for tests. Search the Internet for free screenings and health fairs. Be honest with your doctor about your drinking, smoking, and sexual history. Replacing low estrogen or testosterone; getting your sugar, blood pressure, and cholesterol down; and getting your depression and past issues under control will jump-start your sexuality (and everything else.) **Those who feel good have sex, and those who have sex want to have more sex.** Simple, right?

But it's not so simple to talk to your doctor about sexual things, so I was thrilled to find doctor-authors who directly address the new situations we encounter at midlife. You can photocopy their advice, mark it "confidential," and mail it to the doctor before your appointment if you have a hard time talking about it. *The Wisdom of Menopause, Screaming to Be Heard, The Change Before the Change*, and *Making Love the Way We Used To* are all great resources to copy from, give to your doctor, and say "I was wondering about this." Though they probably should, most internists and family physicians don't ask how your sex life is going; YOU have to bring it up.

What most of us call "estrogen" is actually the hormone estradiol, and it affects every system in your body, from your brain to your veins. The right kind of low-dose birth control can even things out in perimenopause, as described in Chapter 19. When you stop menstruating, your blood levels of estradiol can be brought up to a feeling-good level using bioidentical estradiol in a patch, pill, or cream, balanced with progesterone if you still have your uterus. Vaginal dryness, sleep problems, flashes, aches and pains disappear for most women when they get the bioidentical hormones right. **Recent studies point to patches like Climara and Vivelle as the form of estradiol most likely to restore a woman's sexual desire and touch sensitivity.**

One of the things all the experts say is "use it or lose it " when it comes to vaginal health and sex. The more sex you have, the more sex you *can* have, with an effect similar to strength and mobility gains from weight lifting. In the book *Making Love the Way We Used To…Or Better*, Dr. Alan Altman cautions women not to think that urogenital changes will calm down once the storm of menopause is over. Yes, the body will adjust and hot flashes will eventually go away, but…"**Vaginal dryness and bladder problems do not come from withdrawal of estrogen but from chronic low levels of it.** Without some kind of intervention on your part, the changes will continue, and any symptoms you have will persist and even worsen… Lack of use promotes vaginal atrophy, while frequent intercourse helps maintain elasticity." He describes a forty-eight-year-old patient who had not been sexually active since her divorce five years earlier. She had already begun to lose elasticity, and he informed her that she would have to do something about it now if she wanted to resume sexual activity in the future. Dr Altman recommends penetration of the vagina using your fingers, vaginal dilators, or vibrators to maintain vaginal health, or to **prepare yourself before resuming sex after a time of being without it.** Especially when combined with a regimen of local bioidentical hormones like estriol cream, "using it so you don't lose it" is part of your new fitness program.

Take the local. For those who can't or won't replace estradiol throughout the body, local estrogen replacement in the vaginal area can stop the narrowing of the vagina (vaginal atrophy) and the irritation, inflammation, and painful intercourse. Compounded 0.5mg estriol cream, Vagifem tablets, Estrace cream, and the Estring vaginal ring use bioidentical estradiol to effectively treat vaginal tissue. They can be used along with hormone replacement to keep overall levels relatively low, while symptoms are controlled.

Non-hormonal lubricants like Astroglide and KY Jelly are very trendy these days; KY now has a Warming Liquid that "enhances intimacy" by creating a warm sensation on contact. You can get a booklet on their web site, ky.com, that details new uses of KY by "the girl on the go," such as skin moisturizer and hair gel (but What about Mary?). Some women have good results lubricating with the contents of a liquid Vitamin E capsule. Replens, KY Long Lasting, and Silken Secret take it one step further because they're used to moisturize the vagina regularly (often after a shower) as part of your Midlife Beauty Queen routine, not just before sex.

Kegel exercises are another "use it or lose it" tool for muscle tone around the vagina and opening of the bladder. You may have used these to get back in shape after a pregnancy, and as gravity marches on, you need to resurrect this practice of squeeeeezing the pelvic floor muscles. You'll be ready to stop that urine leak the next time you sneeze, though the unexpected belly laugh will get one past you every once in a while. Locate the muscles by starting and stopping the flow of urine. If you're using your stomach or tush muscles, you're cheating. Put your finger in your vagina and squeeze – now you can feel it. Cross-train with rapid and long squeezes while you brush your teeth and floss, combining good habits. The KegelMaster or Fem-tone Vaginal Weights (shop privately on yahoo.com) will kick it up and up and up a notch.

Midlife changes in men's sexuality— more like cross country than downhill skiing

Midlife men can be the most awesome lovers because they're more knowledgeable about their own response and more mindful of yours. The highly evolved ones are less interested in conquest and putting notches on their gun, and more interested in real intimacy and a sex life that makes sense. (Read about safe sex in Chapter 17.)

Men who lead a healthy life can stay sexually vigorous for a long time. Keeping the weight, blood pressure, and cholesterol down increases blood flow to the erection, and blood flow is what erections are all about. Getting enough sleep increases the human growth hormone in your body, a substance reputed to keep you young. The more muscle mass you have, the more testosterone your body produces. Then there's testosterone's great feedback loop—testosterone makes you desire sex and sex creates more testosterone.

Fruits and vegetables, oatmeal, lean protein, and Omega 3's are the power foods to keep men off the medications that prevent Daddy's Little Helper from coming back for more. (Have you heard why a man gives his penis a name? So he knows what to call the guy who makes most of his decisions.)

SSRI anti-depressants like Prozac, Paxil, and Zoloft; beta-blockers like Inderal; and common drugs like antihistamines, tranquilizers, ulcer meds, and antifungals can cut back on both desire and performance. Erection problems can signal the artery-clogging of heart disease and the nerve damage of diabetes. Living right definitely pays off for Mr. Willy!

Most men don't need extra testosterone, and overdosing can hurt them. Excess testosterone can raise cholesterol, activate prostate cancer, and even promote feminine characteristics. But if blood tests show that testosterone is low, Testim, Androgel or Androderm (patch) are excellent current delivery systems to raise testosterone. Prescription DHEA is another replacement option.

Do women benefit from testosterone replacement? When lack of desire is the problem, a low dose of natural testosterone can be the answer. The level of testosterone in men's products are way too high, so don't even think about sneaking some gel or cutting up a patch from your husband. Dr. Laura Corio, author of *The Change before the Change*, prescribes 2.5 to 5 mg a day of **natural oral micronized testosterone**. In *Women, Weight, and Hormones*, Dr. Vliet starts patients at 1.00 mg of micronized natural testosterone, increasing the dose until you feel better, generally between 2-4 mg. She likes the transdermal cream form, 0.1 mg/gm to 0.4 mg/gm, as well, particularly for women with high cholesterol. She and Dr. Northrup don't recommend Estratest because the estrogens and the testosterone are synthetic, not bioidentical. Vliet's advice is "start low and go slow" with all hormones. A **testosterone patch for women, Intrinsa**, is in the pipeline, and that should be an excellent solution that will be highly publicized.

L-arginine supplement ArginMax for Women showed increased desire in a good study, and the so-called "Barbie

Drug" Melanotan, a synthetic hormone awaiting FDA approval, appears to warm your buns and give you a tan at the same time. (ArginMax for Men and Nutrilite Naturally Together show promise for men.) High-isoflavone shakes from Revival Soy claim to aid energy, sleep, and vaginal moisture. Homeopathic blend Avlimil has a controlled study that shows good results for improving libido and response. Get it delivered monthly less expensively (assess your results during the third month of use). Vaginal oil Zestra dilates blood vessels in the vagina, improving sensation, but the site advises that it's "not the tastiest choice" for oral lovemaking. These non-prescription sex enhancers can be used for fun or to overcome the sexual blahs of depression drugs and other medications.

There are people who just have a low sex drive, and that's okay—as long as they're with a like-minded partner. In a survey, 60% of women answered they'd be happy with cuddling, affection, and no sex. The only problem is, 90% of the men who answered are out looking for the 40% of women who actually want sex! Differences in desire are often compensated for by secret masturbation; he doesn't tell her, she doesn't tell him. That's a good coping mechanism, but why not *tell* the next time you're going to pleasure yourself—tell well, with some juicy details revealing his role in your fantasy? It takes the pressure off your partner, gives him something to think about, or he can jump in.

Another equalizer for out-of-sync sex drives is quickie sex. Quickies are a good antidote for the couple caught in DINS syndrome—dual income, no sex. Men applaud the idea, but are surprised when a woman wants a quickie, wondering what she "gets out of it." She can enjoy a fast and frantic quickie in the shower while the kids are at soccer practice, knowing that he's in the mood. She can feel close and excited, without having to fake an orgasm. On a backyard blanket under the stars, he can make her come without having to perform, saving his excitement for some gourmet sex. The higher-sexed partner is happy, and the other has placed a big deposit in the love bank account, to be withdrawn in some long romantic encounter.

When changes in his erection are the problem, as they are for 50% of men over 50, things can get complicated. More mental, manual, and oral stimulation is often all that's needed for him to get hard and stay hard. Sometimes he can get started, but loses his erection mid-session. You can switch to other forms of lovemaking, or *Sunday Night Sex Show's* Sue Johanson says a cock ring may keep the erection going.

When there's a pattern of problems that stretches for months, the first reaction is usually—"it's stress." They go on a vacation—things still aren't working. She suggests seeing a doctor, he says "Nothing's wrong and talking about it makes it worse." He starts to think, "Maybe it's her," and she starts to wonder too. He stops being affectionate and touching her at all because he doesn't want her to respond and experience failure again. He gets frustrated and withdraws from her; she gets angry and hurt and withdraws from him. This is stupid and unnecessary, people! **A high percentage of erectile dysfunction is due to physical causes**—go to a doctor and find out what they are! Don't fall for the blame game; just emphasize that you're in this together—"Let's go and find out if there's a medical problem because we love each other." Another cause may be emotional issues that can be addressed in couple's therapy.

Men are a lot more willing to go to the doctor since the introduction of Viagra. Take a pill and become the Man of Steel—what could be bad? It may even force him to go for that check-up he's been putting off; do not cooperate with an overweight, out-of-shape hubby who gets Viagra off the internet without a doctor visit. It's effective for about 80% of men who give it a good trial, but may not work for some with high blood pressure or cholesterol, blocked arteries, prostate problems, or out-of-control diabetes. Some men fear the side effects, but doctors have dealt with this drug for quite a while now and can help them ease into it. Women who take Viagra may have better blood flow to the vagina, but results have been mixed. 10,000 men a day get a prescription for Viagra, and that's a lot of erections – but what about their wives?

The Blue Elephant in the Bedroom—Viagra

Because the drug takes an hour or so to work, some Viagra couples may not be able to "sneak up on each other in bed," as they're accustomed to. They have to communicate, make a date with each other, and some women resent the fact that sex is no longer "spontaneous." Others complain that "It's the drug that turns him on, not me." These mindsets bug me; you should thank God such a drug exists, and enjoy the ability to have sex and the extra attention both of you can now lavish on each other as you anticipate sex, instead of blundering into it. Some women will have to check into their own libido or vaginal changes that took place during a period of no sex in the marriage, looking into the therapies discussed above.

During the honeymoon period, when the drug first begins to work and he's excited about it, he may want sex every day (didn't you like to play a lot with a new toy?). A more normal pattern will emerge, and both must practice a little give-and-take (short history of marriage joke: 1968-Niagara. 2000-Viagra). Women who've worked hard to accept their sexless marriage have to have some time to adjust to the new reality. Some Viagra couples will find they've swept relationship problems under the rug while dealing with the erections, and they've got to heal their feelings for one another. Mr. Viagra will have to be patient, seduce his wife, and become a better lover to bring her interest back, while she needs to reassure him that she wants to be with him, but may need some time. If he can depend on his erection, he can spend more time on foreplay and not worry about "losing it." You can light the candles and warm up the massage oil again, and both can spend time caring for each other—before, during, and after lovemaking. Eventually he may regain the confidence he lost and not even need the drug, or he'll take better care of himself so he can continue to use it without worrying about his health.

The Checklist

❑ I. 20 million Viagra prescriptions have changed over-40 sex forever, and new drugs are on the scene. Levitra is reported to have a more rapid "onset of action" and doesn't need to be taken on an empty stomach like Viagra. Cialis, dubbed "the weekender," will reintroduce some spontaneity because its effects are said to last 36 hours, though it can't be taken every day.

❑ 2. The vagina is self-cleansing; there is no medical need to douche. If you have chronic discharge, use a mild, disposable vinegar-and-water douche from the supermarket no more than twice a week. Also use this if you need to cleanse Prochieve gel (used in hormone replacement) before lovemaking. Stay out of public hot tubs if you have a tendency toward irritation.

❑ 3. Tell your guy—it's estimated that for every 35 lbs of extra weight you lose, you get one more inch of visible penis. Of course, he'll also feel sexier if he's looking good!

❑ **4.** It's best to be completely frank and include lots of details in a sex book. That's what makes *Sex Over 50* by Susan Bakos and therapist Joel Block such a great book—they include details about everything from how to get better at oral to what's normal as time goes by. Sue Johanson, the Canadian "sex lady" on the *Sunday Night Sex Show* covers everything from boredom to bondage in her book *Sex, Sex, and More Sex. How to Be a Great Lover* and *How to Give Her Absolute Pleasure* detail Lou Paget's explicit sexpertise, including the Ode to Bryan. For steamy stories, check out Lonnie Barbach's *Seductions: Tales of Erotic Persuasion* or books by Joan Elizabeth Lloyd.

❑ **5.** Sources of sexual stuff that don't sell your name to other companies include the Adam and Eve Catalogue and Good Vibrations, adameve.com and goodvibes.com. Don't go wandering around the Internet unless you want to start receiving weird pop-ups and mail.

The Checkup from the Neck Up

❑ When it's time for lovemaking, I am totally present, into my lover and not thinking about other things.

❑ I accept that my body is the best it can be right now, and feel confident and attractive, knowing that enjoyment and enthusiasm are the sexiest qualities.

❑ We have reorganized our lives to make time for sex, and we've fired up our time in the bedroom by firing up our lives!

❑ I tell my lover what I need in the right way and at the right time, and he can trust me to hear and accept his needs without judging him.

15.

What Goes Around Comes Around—
It may be your turn to be Mom & Dad to Mom & Dad.

"Some people might say, Who would want to be 90? And I say, Anyone who is 89."
—**Phyllis Diller** on "Larry King Live"

Have you really talked to your parents lately? In the whiz-bang of holidays and life, have you taken the time to hear their stories of childhood, the war years, courtship, work, and what life was like when they were your age? Summer days, long drives, and waiting in doctor's offices seem to be the best settings for these conversations. I've seen them come alive, telling their successes and silly mistakes with fresh insight after seeing a period movie that brought it all rushing back for them. These stories are precious, they are your legacy, and if your children are too young or self-absorbed right now to listen, you must save it for them.

After you've listened to the good stuff, you may be entitled to hear the bad stuff. Ask specific questions relating to the nuances you picked up along the way. "Mom, no one seems to have anything good to say about your father. Can you remember anything about that?" "Your sister/brother was so much older than you. Do you think you grew up differently than she/he did?" The big question, perhaps appropriate to ask after an illness, is something wide-open like "Is there something you always wanted to tell me, but you didn't want to bother me with it?" You have to be strong to handle that answer, but the gift may be that it reveals a hidden agenda that shaped you.

Take my parents—PLEASE!

Today's seniors are often caught up in lots of activities, travel, work, and socializing, and barely have time to worry about what you're doing. But many people have to deal with difficult, strong-willed parents who act like immature kids. They offer personal and financial advice without observing proper boundaries, using guilt and other unfair tactics. You may absorb it and let it build up until—BOOM!—you freak out, blow up, and ruin some holiday or special occasion because you just can't take it anymore. Start a grown-up relationship now with some strategies.

- Limit the information you reveal to them. There are some things your parents just won't handle well.
- Include Mom in your book group or Dad in your husband's weekly card game, volunteer at the library together, or have them sub for you in doing something with the kids. Have them teach the family how to play canasta, so you have something to do on holidays other than talk about sensitive topics. You'll see a whole new side of them in a different setting or activity.
- Let them know good and bad times to call—they're not

mind readers. Establish regular times and holidays to catch up and fill in the gaps with e-mail or funny cards.

- Stop expecting them to repair the damage from the past. It's your job to accept and move on now, you're a big girl. Keep the connection alive through good times and bad so you have no regrets down the road.

Bad behavior may just be crankiness or—if it seems really over the top—it may be the beginning of Alzheimer's disease. Families tend to ignore the subtle beginnings of the disease, thinking that the irritability and poor judgment are just normal aging. That's bad because Aricept, Reminyl, and Exelon, the medications that slow the disease's progress, work best in the early stages. Simple ibuprofen and naproxen break up the brain plaque of the disease. Here's a list of early warning signs from a dementia specialist, Dr. Rodman Shankle, the kind of doctor you should see for your parent's evaluation:

- recent memory loss that affects job skills
- difficulty performing familiar tasks
- problems with language
- disorientation of time and place
- poor or decreased judgment
- problems with abstract thinking
- misplacing things
- changes in mood or behavior
- changes in personality
- loss of initiative

Author Jacqueline Marcell quotes this list and provides many other resources in her book *Elder Rage*, where she tells the funny and frustrating true story of her struggle with her ailing parents. She also provides loads of practical info like how to get an elder to give up driving and how to successfully navigate the maze of elder care.

Vitamin Xercise – the best anti-ager at any age!
Sometimes heart rate and blood pressure don't tell the whole
story; your parent just doesn't seem right to you. Can they rise
from a chair without using their arms? Are they shuffling
unsteadily instead of walking? After you've ruled out drug
interactions, a good course of action is some individual
counseling on exercise. Working on balance, strength,
mobility, and flexibility can really help seniors to stay
independent. Since home programs aren't often covered by
Medicare, **maybe you can help your parent adapt the
outpatient physical therapy program they qualified for**.
Physical therapists are usually willing to help you facilitate the
home program, knowing how effective that can be in
preventing falls and other problems. Miriam Nelson's books —
Strong Women Stay Young; Strong Women, Strong Bones and
others—have excellent, very simple programs you can help
your parent use or adapt at home.

Videos or a class are really the best investment for seniors
looking to get strong and healthy. If you can find an
appropriate class, it's also a great social opportunity, combating
the isolation of many older adults. Failing that, a very targeted
video is *Geri Fit*, with instructor Francesca Gern, designed by a
geriatrician and getting as much as 800% results in strength
gain! For variety, mix in *Richard Simmons and the Silver Foxes*
and Leslie Sansone's *Walk and Fit for Older Adults*. I can't think
of a better birthday or Mother's Day gift to try out together.

What's wrong with me today?
Maybe your elder seems constantly to have health crises
that turn out to be nothing. This can be a sign of depression
that can be helped with counseling and medication. But
sometimes it's a given each time you're on the phone with

them; they've just eaten something "bad" or discovered a new set of symptoms that may represent some weird disease. They've discovered that your love and brain chemistry seem only directed at them when they're sick, so they find ways to get their love jolts by waking up in the morning and saying, "What's wrong with me today?" Of course, the "been there" attitude will prevail after awhile, and you will stop responding to the latest illness, and your loved one.

Make a decision to continue relating by responding only to any other issue they bring up. When I called my mother and she would describe her urinary and bowel patterns in excruciating detail, I would barely respond. When she mentioned *anything else*—a nurse's kindness, a friend's visit—I responded with interest and enthusiasm. In person, I would only meet her eyes and respond when she talked about *anything else*. After a time, our conversations veered away from toileting toward other things. In midlife you must realize that people have "been there and done that" with *your* conversational ticks too, so you must find creative ways to continue to pay attention to Mom and Dad.

Mom or Dad's "new friend"

Sometimes parents remarry later in life or have a "new friend." In an article in *More* magazine titled "I Have a Wicked Stepmother", the anonymous author notes that her father's friend Phyllis was sweet when they were dating, but the fangs were bared immediately after the honeymoon. Phyllis gave everything that had belonged to her mother to the cleaning lady when she moved into her father's house and put away all the pictures of the kids and grandkids. Her Dad seemed barely interested in his family, absorbed as he was in his new round of card games and golf lessons.

A friend of mine tells similar horror stories of Dad asking the daughter-in-law for a ring he'd given her after Mom died; he wanted to give it to the new wife! The couple began their travels around the world, bringing back a tissue box from a famous hotel as a souvenir for the grandkids! (You know it's a true story because I couldn't make that up.)

I remember a younger man my mother hooked up with about a year after my Dad died. All of a sudden, Mom bought a waterbed and wore tight jeans and high heels. She was so happy and excited! Right after the alcohol in their lifestyle started conflicting with her medication and her health, his ex-wife called, looking for her alimony and child support. Mom's "new friend" disappeared almost immediately.

Focus on the good qualities of the new partner, stop trying to change the relationship, and learn the true meaning of "grin and bear it." If someone throws down the argument glove, don't pick it up. Just be glad they have someone to share their life with.

People seem to go one way or the other as they get into their 70's and beyond—either more combative and grouchy, or totally nonconfrontational and timid. You wonder why they fly off the handle so easily or why they don't stand up to the mate who's bullying them. It seems that they either want passionately to be "right" or they just want to peacefully go with the flow. Just remember that you were a grouchy, demanding, unpredictable little pooper once yourself, so now it's time to pay your dues.

The Checklist

❏ I. For those in retirement, *Streetwise Retirement Planning* looks at annuities, IRAs, Medicare, Social Security and other concerns; provides assessment tools; and details how to counter medical crises, market fluctuations, and other surprises.

❏ 2. Check for possible drug and herbal interactions on drugdigest.org. A copy of the *Merck Manual* is nice to have.

❏ 3. For the senior in need of interaction, going to the Senior Center for the first time is very nerve-wracking. Ask them to call and reassure her or stop by for a tour after you've been out to lunch. *The Complete Eldercare Planner* is a good guide for caregivers.

❏ 4. Read cautions and advice on planning a funeral at funerals.org. Be appalled by funeral scams on funerals-ripoffs.org.

The Checkup from the Neck Up

❏ As adult daughters, we can understand and affirm our parents more than ever.

❏ I am always working toward forgiveness, intimacy, and mutual respect; I enjoy the good and let go of the bad.

❏ Being right is the booby prize; being happy is the gift we strive for together.

❏ I wait for the right moment to talk about disability, long-term care and last wishes, but we will have the conversations we need to have.

16.

Friends Help You Love Your Life—
Be the model of the best friend you'd like to have!

"To succeed in any intimate relationship, you need a certain freedom to fail. Most experts at friendship have gone through a few ruptured relationships and realize that it will happen occasionally. They do their best to maintain their friendships and family connections, but if something goes wrong, they do not automatically assume that something is wrong with them. Friendships, like plants, can die naturally. People move away from each other in interests and needs. There is a certain attrition in all things. Lifelong relationships may be wonderful, but they are quite rare. When we have had a good friendship for a few months or a few years, we should be grateful for the time we had together rather than lamenting that it did not last forever."
—The Friendship Factor, **Alan Loy McGinnis**

Though you may feel hurt or numb by the actions of old friends, resolve to open your heart to new relationships. New friends are not in your home, and especially <u>not</u> on your

TV. You may be tired from chauffeuring kids, juggling the job, and running your household, but being out in the big world is central to your growth as a person and the length of your holiday card list. In order to have more friends, you have to be out at school or community events, weekend festivals—anywhere but in your home. Start a conversation at the soccer game by asking, "Which one is your son?" Hang around after your class and get to know someone. Introduce yourself to the new person at work. When you're out shopping, talk to the person next to you.

Find friends who share your values and make the kinds of choices you would make.
I'd rather not spend a lot of time around women who criticize their husbands, label their children, and talk about soap operas, and Scott is not big on guys who talk about guns, getting wasted, and going to strip clubs. You may walk into a group where the topics are along those lines, but some of those people are wonderful to talk to privately. I'm not saying your friends should be *like you*; instead, they should expand your ideas about what choices are available and how to joyfully do the right thing.

Share your life with encouragers who are transparent, yet know how to keep a secret. We all have friends and family who keep up the façade of perfection. They're uncomfortable when people get real. They don't like it when you "do your dirty laundry" and share a challenge, probably because it looks a lot like *their* dirty laundry. When you share something difficult, they can't relate; when you share something great, they tell you they've always had that or done it that way. Well, yaaahoo for them, but I'd rather share my stories with someone who trusts me by sharing mistakes, burdens, and whether this dress makes me look like a parade float. And I need to know that whatever I share in confidence will stay that way – no matter what!

In addition to control freaks, watch out for:

- **people who use you as a garbage can with a hairy lid.** Your complaining buddies say things like "We just can't win, can we? Why bother?" If you're guilty of this, start to set a good example by discovering what's positive in situations and set a personal limit on whining. I know it feels good to release that venom, but if people start finding ways to leave the room when you enter, it's time to decline the whining! I can hunker down and feel part of the group by griping, but I can also strive to find something to celebrate instead. Share problems and possible solutions in the same conversation. Tell your high maintenance friend (high on demand, low on supply) "The next time we get together, let's not talk about so-and-so," (her ex's new girlfriend).

- **dream destroyers. "Yes, you could go to law school, but the field is so crowded, isn't it?"** This is fear and doubt talking, and it's never valuable to be the killjoy. Encourage or be silent. Both are very powerful. Don't share your dreams with people who haven't supported you in the past. I have friends who enjoy my company, but I can't count on them and I know they think the positive attitudes in this book are nauseating. Try to share deep feelings only with someone who is on your wavelength in the attitude department.

- **manipulators. "Dad would feel so uncomfortable with someone he doesn't know taking care of him, and with all he's done for you…"** Putting your whole self into your midlife pursuits shouldn't happen at the expense of your sanity. Strive for balance and ask for

help in a way that doesn't accuse or bring up the past.
Confess your shortcomings—"I know I haven't done as
much as you have"—but define your boundaries as
well. State what you can do from this point forward,
and list what else needs to be done by someone else.
When you hear that phrase that causes you to lose
control, say, "I understand that you feel that way, but we
really need to find a new solution." You'd probably be
justified in freaking out when somebody comes up with
the same old line, but where will it get you? "Assertive,
effective, and fair" are the new words you use to
describe yourself.

Big girls know how to set boundaries and say no. If your
friends always bring their unruly kids to adult parties, tell them
"I hope you can get a sitter and join us." If they ask for a loan,
either give it and don't expect it back, or say, "I'm sorry, this
just isn't a good time for me." If they always expect your
professional services without pay, explain that your schedule is
full right now, but "down the road I'll definitely give you the
'friends' discount." Be charitable and forgiving—your shared
history and good times are worth much more than these
annoyances, and you may have to decide the friendship is just
worth the weirdo tendencies.

Girls just wanna have fun times together.

Healthy parents provide opportunities for kids to explore
and grow. It's hard to let go, but you get through the first
slumber party, the talent show, two weeks at camp, and that
really long night of the prom. When they fail, we die a little,
remembering times when *we* tried and failed. When things go
well, we rejoice in their new skills and friendships.

At midlife, we have to provide those growth opportunities for ourselves if we want to stay juicy and young. **How about starting a playgroup?** People who have a little more time plan both outies and innies for the rest of the group. What's an innie? That's where you get together in someone's house and play bunko, discuss a book, or exercise together. A generous fellow exerciser hosts a holiday cookie exchange every year in her beautifully decorated home. My local Newcomers and Friends group provides opportunities like this, including day and evening book groups and coffees with and without kids. How about a sleepover with your sisters or sisters-in-law? An outtie is going to the theatre or a museum exhibition, attending a lecture, or volunteering at a soup kitchen together. Clear the date, and go for it!

Have a slumber party! Fun, crazy times, and stupid things to laugh about are the cornerstones of friendship. Priscilla and I will always remember the panty exchange we had at my slumber party a few years ago. Everyone had to bring a wrapped pair of panties to put in a bag in the middle of our pajama circle. One by one, we hammed it up as we pulled out outrageous panties with flags, animal prints, and beads. Of course, the shyest, most subdued woman there got the glitziest thong panty with feathers!

After a meal of pizza and salad, we shared popcorn and cut-up fruit while being transported to California's Napa Valley with *A Walk in the Clouds*, a love story/chick flick extraordinaire. Some fell asleep in Rugrats sleeping bags borrowed from their kids, while others traded stories into the wee hours. My husband (good sport) whipped up veggie omelets Saturday morning, and a bunch of wired women hit the road in their minivans, streaking toward soccer games and business commitments with a new enthusiasm born of friendship. I've experienced two "retreats," where a generous friend offers her cabin for a weekend and sharing, eating, giggling and movie-watching lead to a friendly uplift for all attendees. Complaining and criticizing are kept on the constructive side. Sharing serious problems can be done in private, with someone who can handle it.

Whether it's planning a theatre outing, a day at the beach, or a simple lunch, creating memories with friends takes time and planning. If you don't put it on the calendar, you won't do it. My mom sniffed at the neighbors who got together for coffee and conversation. She spent the time making her home spotless and her garden lush. When my dad died and she needed that support system, it wasn't there. A little coffee klotching is a good thing and an investment into a happier future.

Friendship can be complicated. At the Matisse/Picasso exhibit touring the country in 2003, the lifelong rivalry of these two giants was revealed as their paintings were exhibited side by side. Supposedly they criticized and disliked one another, but you could see very plainly that each artist grew from watching the other. Alluding to each other's work with bits of pattern and similar subjects, their competition was fierce. Through the years and two world wars, their rivalry turned to respect. In the end, they lived near each other in the south of France and saw each other often. When Matisse died, Picasso said, "I continue his work."

Don't give up on friendship. Yes, life evolves and your friend moves away, marries somebody you can't stand, falls out of touch, and doesn't return the reply card for your big birthday party. You may always have been the person maintaining the relationship, and you feel hurt that she never reciprocates. She may communicate only via e-mail, while you like to call. Continue to forgive and don't forget what was special about the two of you. **Don't obsess, but every once in a while put an**

opportunity out there for your old friend to pick up the ball.
I had a lovely surprise recently when an old friend who'd gone
through a divorce finally responded to years of cards and e-mails.
No, she hadn't cancelled out everyone in her old life; she was
just "busy." When we thought about it, we realized she'd
always been that way, flying off to the next exciting installment
of her life without bothering to tidy up the details from the last.
**Bottom line—if you sow good friendship practices, you'll
reap great friendships and you will eventually reap what you
sow, even if you don't reap *when* you sow.** If you cultivate
the thick skin that repels hurt feelings and the thin heart that
welcomes intimacy, interesting people will surround you.
Friendship is vitally important in midlife as families and life
change, so we need to get better at getting and keeping friends.

In particular, it's important to seek out and honor older
women. They're farther down the road, closer to knowing
what we're on this earth to do. When they've sage-ed instead
of aged, they've already purged meaningless things from their
lives and stopped distracting themselves with go-nowhere
pastimes. If young women are the buds, older women are the
blossoms. Let them pour out their wisdom and show us how to
grow more beautiful and more joyful. Yes, your mother can
stop acting motherly all the time and be your best friend.

**Enough with the beauty contest—stop commenting on
every woman who walks in the room!** Let's face it—when we
make negative statements about people behind their backs, we
get a little power jolt out of it. But in truth, the only thing
we're reflecting is our own insecurity, our own powerless,
unworthy self-concept. If you don't have the courage to talk
directly with the person you have a problem with, stash the
assassination attempt. And didn't your mother tell you to
watch out for friends who gossip, 'cause the next friend they'll

gossip about is you? (Personally, I never gossip, but I can give you the names of certain people who do.) When you skunk the place up with stinking words, someone will get wind of it and come back 'atcha.

Imagine if you just made your home, your cubicle at work, your car, and your mouth a positive, gossip-free zone. Change the only person you can change, and that's you. When a whisper fest gets started while you're standing there, get busy with a task you just remembered. Make yourself so busy building your dreams, you have no time to tear down others'. When the poisonous snakes and frogs aren't flying out of your mouth, there's plenty of room for diamonds and flowers to flow out instead.

The Checklist

❏ For chick-flicks beyond the obvious (*Pretty Woman, Working Girl, Dirty Dancing, My Big Fat Greek Wedding,* and *Miss Congeniality*) you might think about oldies but goodies: *Some Like It Hot, All About Eve, Breakfast At Tiffany's, Woman of the Year, Theodora Goes Wild, Madame X*

❏ "Transformation" movies*: Moonstruck, Private Benjamin, Married to the Mob, Funny Girl, Funny Face, Never Been Kissed, A Star is Born*

❏ Midlife*: Summertime, Shirley Valentine, Saving Grace, Peggy Sue Got Married, The Secret Life of Girls, Music of the Heart, Calendar Girls, Something's Gotta Give*

Other women's get-together ideas:

❏ Go to un-finishing school and learn how to be girls again instead of women—learn rowing, mountain biking, surfing, motorcycle riding, or other "unladylike" sports.

❏ Go the ultra-chick root—cooking clubs, quilting bees, needlework "stitch & bitch" sessions, greeting card-making, belly-dancing, learning massage, dance lessons, perfume testing, cookie decorating, makeup and facials, ice-cream sundae bar with all the fixings, mashed potato bar (cheddar, bacon, salmon, olives?).

❏ If you can't get together in person, how about instant messaging at a certain time each week/month, or group e-mail? Girlfriends can hop on and add their two cents any old time.

Use the new Book Browser on barnesandnoble.com to come up with lists of mysteries, romances, best sellers, or whatever for your book group or check *The Readers' Choice* or *The Reading Group Book* for recommendations with provocative discussion questions. For suggestions beyond the obvious *The Lovely Bones* and *The Red Tent*, read the quirky *Booked* site, cynthiacrossen.com.

17 .

Soaring Solo
Living Large with a Side of Guys

"Life is what happens to you while you are making other plans."
—**Lily Tomlin**

"Sometimes I wonder if men and women really suit each other. Perhaps they should live next door and just visit now and then"
—**Katherine Hepburn**

Most women (70%) will be single at some point in their lives. We're marrying later, divorcing more often, and outliving our husbands by years, and sometimes by *decades*. Cobbling together a back-up system of friends, family, and colleagues has been or will be a key task. **Support systems beyond marriage are being slapped together and have been celebrated by every sitcom from The Golden Girls to The Gilmore Girls.**

The support system single moms dream about is to get a wife! Wouldn't it be great to have that idealized version of a wife, that person who joyfully supports your life and career by taking care of all the nitty-gritty details? In your working life, they call this person your assistant, at home it's the nanny or the housekeeper, but you would have to hire a staff of 3 or 4 to do what wives really do out of love—everything! Single women, and especially single moms, struggle with the lack of a partner. In *Flying Solo, Single Women in Midlife*, authors Anderson and Stewart recognize the sheer volume of the problem:

"The responsibility of handling every single chore, making every decision, large and small, on one's own, can spoil women's ability to feel like carefree pilots soaring above the clouds. Instead, they end up feeling like frantic air-traffic controllers trying to avoid the collision of several jumbo jets…Spontaneity is a paradise lost; 'going with the flow,' a laughable concept. Organization, precision, and endless forethought are the necessary staples…dealing responsibly with money, especially in relation to long-term planning, is the final frontier of their independence. Even when single women are soaring freely above the clouds of life's routine tasks, dealing with their own financial issues can feel like flying into the heart of a treacherous storm. They rarely crash, but the ride can be rough and frightening."

This whole thing about becoming a bag lady is especially prevalent among single women, and a divorced woman with a child is nearly three times more likely to file for bankruptcy than a single person with no children. Even high-earning women fear that they'll lose it all and mumble to themselves while sleeping on newspapers in the subway. There's a deep insecurity, a fear of doing something wrong, a guilty conviction that somehow we're not entitled to be first-class financial citizens. Maybe we fear that if we take responsibility for our finances, Prince Charming won't come along and take care of us. Hell-o-o, the Prince has left the building! Even the most prince-like guys need partnering and mutual effort in today's crazy, uncertain economy. Money-competent women who take responsibility for their financial futures exude the same confidence that sexually aware women do, and they can be man-magnets for that very reason.

Today's single Midlife Mama is likely to say "I'd love a great long-term relationship with someone, but you won't catch me washing his socks!" With changes in women's incomes and the percentages of people touched by divorce came a new attitude about singledom, particularly for the over-45 crowd. Our massively educated generation of women will find only three single men to every ten single women who've been through college. Men with money tend to "pull a Michael Douglas," marry a younger woman, and start over. That leaves fewer men who are educated and/or have money on the playing field. So what's a woman who wants some male company to do?

- **Be out and about in groups or pairs**, and have the next outing planned when you go to this one. For example, when you go to a singles event at church, know where the next birthday party, karaoke evening, lecture, or singles' service opportunity is planned so you and your friends can invite groups of men to join you.

- **Find something to compliment about everyone you meet** ("Rachael tells me you're a real star at work"), but make stronger eye contact with men you're interested in. Practice until you're comfortable with it; eye contact and a smile make men in a crowd know you're approachable. Yes, I know this feels contrived. But you have to find some way to let lookers know you're looking too.

- **Listen intensely**. Keep sarcasm and complaining out of your speech. Relate and reassure, saying things like "These get-togethers are interesting, aren't they?" with a smile. Sharing the humor in uncomfortable introductions puts everyone at ease.

- **Don't be afraid of some of the new trends in dating.**
You may not want to be on TV's *Blind Date or A Dating
Story*—with all the world watching your smooth dating
moves—but finding your old high school flame might
be worthwhile. Find Mr. First Kiss using a plain old
directory like switchboard.com or whitepages.com, a
search engine like Google, or a high school reunion site
like classmates.com or reunion.com. **Favorite faith-
based sites are eharmony.com "to find your Christian
soul mate" and JDate.com for Jewish singles.**

- **Another new trend is speed dating**, a romantic round
robin where you sit across from up to 30 "dates" and
talk for a few minutes until the bell rings and you move
on to the next one. Only when both speeders fill out
"yes" on their dance cards do phone numbers get
exchanged. Hurry to speeddating.com (Jewish singles)
or hurrydate.com.

- **Don't head into cyber-, print personal, or speed-
dating without a guide**—*Cast Your Net*, by Eric Fagan.
He details the top sites (kiss, match, or date.com
among them), how to present your "fun loving" self in
the best light, **safety issues**, and "red flag" questions to
ask that save time and heartache.

- **Don't bet on the Prince**, only dating men who meet
certain requirements. Yes, it's important to have a vision
of the kind of man you want, but that sweet spirit may
be hiding under a bald head or an ethnicity you know
nothing about; take the blinders off and don't worry
about what your friends might think.

- **Call every human being you know** and ask them to fix
you up. Of those currently married, 50% were
introduced by friends or family.

- **Break out of the comfort zone of certain bars and restaurants** and go to different places with different friends if you want different results. Be the person laughing the most and you'll attract people who want to laugh.

Your midlife love doesn't have to have the same structure and intent as your original love. When you find someone special, you can love to be together sometimes or all the time, fitting in your old framework or creating a new or extra one, gulping life together or feeding it to one another in tiny, elegant bits of time. You can talk on the phone or instant messaging for hours; reserve long weekends, vacations, and holidays for each other; or do a same-time-next weekend thing. You can support each other personally and professionally while doing each other's laundry and dishes…or not. You can prepare to leave for the restaurant while pondering his repeated question "Where's my…" or not. You can always find your leftover Thai noodle dish waiting for you in the frig…or not.

The question you have to ask yourself is, "Can I live with the boundaries of a limited relationship?" If you're always wondering who else he's seeing during the week, definitely not. If you're met with silence or irritation when you talk about 'changing the deal,' probably not. If you've known each other over a year, he knows your family, but you haven't been introduced to his—no way.

Martha and Richard found each other through a personal ad, and from the moment they met they wanted to spend all their time together. "We never looked at any option except getting married and living together 24/7," she says, now married for seven years. Their grown families merge pleasantly on occasion, but mostly it's just the two of them looking after each other. The lesson? Relationships with lots of boundaries are great, but if you want the traditional model of two people who are intensely close, keep looking until you find someone who feels the same way. They're out there, if you're willing to look.

Is there just one "soul mate" out there for you, and anyone else is just settled-for? Do you have a romantic destiny, and you've either already experienced it or you're still looking? I don't think so. There are hundreds of potential partners out there for you, and the perfect cosmic union doesn't exist. In Christian and Jewish religious traditions, marriage is holy and the couple can ask God for help and guidance, but responsibility for making the relationship work is squarely on our own shoulders. That's a relief for midlife couples who have compatibility and passion—one less thing to worry about. The midlife Attitude of Gratitude, thankfulness for every small comfort and bit of happiness, should lead us away from loneliness and seeking perfection and toward feeling whole in ourselves, while also seeking connection.

One of the most bewildering aspects of being single today is sex. Is "Sex and the City" the new model, or do the old rules still hold? When interviewed, the stars of S & TC say they have never and would never have the promiscuous, random sex depicted on the show even if they could, so what does that tell you? Still, the desire to be transported, carried away, and spontaneous is a persistent theme on the wish lists of midlife women. Ex-hippies who participated in the 70's sexual revolution go back to the mindset of those days without acknowledging that the situation has completely changed.

Midlife women I interviewed confessed to having sex on the third date, less than five weeks into the relationship, and having sex without condoms shortly after that. Many didn't know that you could get diseases from the pre-ejaculate fluid of oral sex. A surprising number had sex on vacation with a relative stranger. (Talk about a vacation to die for.) My question is, if he's done that with you, what do you think he's done with those who preceded you? How much credibility does your sexual history have with him if you've moved quickly, and how desperate do you look? How many women have found out they weren't "the only one" when the test was positive and it was too late? "I have to trust him," "I'm afraid he'll move on," "He seems healthy," and "He says he can't come using those," are some of the excuses I heard. (See more in The Checklist.) Girlfriends, it always comes down to the same thing, doesn't it? You have to love yourself enough to make the right choices!

Some health-oriented single friends of mine describe this scenario: " I won't have sex with a man I've clicked with until I've known him at least three months, we've been together in various settings, and I've seen him in context, where he lives, his friends, hopefully some family. We use condoms for the first six months that we're intimate, and after that we share AIDS test results." Spontaneous and sizzlingly sexy? No. Smart? Seems so. The new OraQuick Rapid HIV-1 Antibody Test, recently approved by the FDA, requires one drop of blood and delivers results in 20 minutes. You'll find home tests on the Internet you mail, wait three days, and get your results on an 800-number.

While it may no longer be important for you to pursue "The Dream"—marriage and a family—it is very important to have a new dream, a plan of action for getting what you want. Change is inevitable, but the choices you make should help you feel powerful and define what you really want. Don't be paralyzed and afraid to fail. Create a personal safety net and invest time in yourself.

The Checklist

More excuses not to use condoms and their answers beyond "No glove, no love, Baby":

I can't feel anything when I wear a condom—With a condom, we'll both relax, and an infection doesn't feel good either.

I'll lose my erection—I'll help you put it on; that'll help you stay hard.

Trust me, I love you, real men don't—A real man who cares about me will help us to protect ourselves from infections we may not realize we have.

You carry condoms?—I felt passionate about you, and I care about both of us.

The Checkup from the Neck Up

❑ Being single gives me many opportunities to learn new things and get better at managing all aspects of my life.

❑ I use my freedom and flexibility to expand my life.

❑ I live fully and honestly, enjoying new experiences; if someone decides to share my life, that'll be great.

❑ Dating is uncomfortable for him too, so I need to be kind, clear, and true to my own strengths and weaknesses.

18.

Anything Worth Doing is Worth Doing Now!
Sail around the world, open an inn, become a minister, change careers?

"We'd love our bodies to be wild, our hearts to be carefree, our awareness of consequences to be nonexistent. As adults we're expected to tolerate ungratifying work, mortgages, and unreasonable bosses…No wonder we want to run away to sea or try another sexual partner. You're afraid your ability to be amazed will soon be gone forever…Your restlessness is telling you that the time has come to reclaim your personality and your originality and your joy at simply being alive, to become an explorer once again…"
—It's Only Too Late If You Don't Start Now, **Barbara Sher**

The bank manager chucked it all to counsel minority business owners. The Internet whiz kid is now the chief exec at a disaster-relief agency. The ESPN sportscaster became a teacher and girls' basketball coach in a Catholic middle school. High-powered, high-tech entrepreneurs from the 90's show off water purifiers, solar collectors, and leg-powered irrigation pumps designed to improve life in the third world and make their own lives more meaningful.

Demographers call this trend "downshifting"—**trading higher paychecks for more free time, joy, and significance.** A 2002 survey of Fortune 1000 executives found that 54% did *not* aspire to become chief executive of their company, compared with 26% the year before. Many women who have broken through the glass ceiling have discovered they don't like the air up there, and decided instead to pursue balance and meaning in their lives. **Let's not dismiss it as a "midlife crisis" or a "Mom thing."** Many polls have shown that only a small percentage of these job shifters have small children at home, men lag only 10% behind women in their search for simplicity, and young people right out of college now ask interviewers about work-life balance.

What are your natural talents and abilities and how can you apply them to something you'd *like* to do? This step is important, especially if you've just fallen into whatever floated by in the past. Imagine what it would be like doing your current job with different people; maybe you just need the same field with different colleagues. Have you talked to people about what it takes to succeed in the field you're looking at? Knowing that your dreams of a great working life are God's gift to you, that working toward your dreams will enrich everyone you love, and that dreams help you love your life, ask yourself…

• **What was I doing when I last "lost all track of time"?** Gardening, singing, designing a web site?

• **Where would I go and what would I do if I were lucky,** if I were someone I admire, if I could magically have a certain talent, if I were invisible, if I were a man, if I couldn't fail, if I didn't have to fit into others' lives, if I could start anywhere and live anywhere, if money wasn't a consideration?

• **What job would I do for free?** What do people say I'm very good at?

- **Someone gives me a million dollars**, and I have to spend it on myself. **Where would I go and what would I buy?** Write it all down, no matter how "ridiculous." What worthwhile people and projects would I donate money and time to, if I could?

- **What would my perfect regular working (not vacation) day look like?** What would I be doing, who would I be with, what would my surroundings be like? Why does this work feel so great and why would I get so much money and/or satisfaction for doing it?

- **What would I tell my grandkids I'm most proud of ?** How do I want to be remembered?

Most people spend more time planning their annual vacation than they spend mapping out the rest of their lives. The classic books in this field are *What Color is Your Parachute?* and *Do What You Are*, but for midlife, I like *The Pathfinder: How to Choose or Change Your Career for a Lifetime of Satisfaction and Success.* Author Nicholas Lore will fully engage you in the process of getting off autopilot. There's a very special book for artists who want to tap into their creativity—*The Artist's Way*, by Julia Cameron. She has a unique perspective on the creative process, using a "Morning Pages" structured journal-writing program that identifies your special viewpoint and the blocks, toxic relationships, and fears that are holding you back. Again, **you empower yourself by believing your life is worth the time to discover and move forward with what you really want to do.**

Filling in for those who are downshifting or dropping out entirely are those who've been working in flexible jobs or at home, but want to spend *more* time at the office and **kick their careers up a notch.** You can join the women at the top of American companies, many of them midlife career changers who started in traditional "women's" positions: Carly Fiorina at Hewlett Packard; Betsy Holden at Kraft Foods; e-Bay's Meg Whitman; and Anne Mulcahy of Xerox. I'm sure you're aware that there is a double standard for men and women in some professions; Barbara Walters was a "wise older woman" of TV at 50, while Dan Rather at 50 was the "young guy" who replaced Walter Cronkite. Be aware, but don't let perception hold you back.

Be the CEO of YOU

For practical, git-down-and-do-it details on the job hunt, read *Women for Hire*. This book will bring you up to date on networking, how to use the Internet, and hundreds of upbeat strategies on finding a job. The authors know the areas where women are generally weak, and they give you the insider information you need to proceed with confidence.

Learn how to do informational interviews and network; this is the one area women are most ignorant and fearful of. This comes from the part of us that fears to ask for what we need. When you're negotiating salary, act like the grownups. Check ads for positions like yours on the Internet, with employment agencies, and trade publications. Know your target and bottom numbers when you walk in, but don't reveal them until you're talking to someone who can actually hire you. Use phrases like "What sort of flexibility do you have?" and "What did you have in mind?" Give a ridiculously high figure that makes everyone laugh, and then ask "If half-a-mill isn't right, what *did* you have in mind? Make them talk first. Once you get that new job, don't get comfortable; you should always be networking with an eye on your *next* job!

Know your strengths, and watch the help wanted ads on Sundays for employers who need what you have. You'll begin to see the types of companies you might move to, and you can study the trends in those industries. If the mortgage business is collapsing, look at health care. If you're selling in a dying industry, get retrained for a growing industry. Learn how to do PowerPoint or specialty data bases, get a certification or licensed training—you probably won't earn back the cost of another degree after 40.

Promote yourself as offering a lot of bang for the buck because of your hard-earned experience. Did some young thang get a division through the last recession, or did you? Break out your huge Rolodex/Palm list of contacts in your industry; how many 25-year-olds have that? Flaunt the fact that you're an empty nester—with no soccer games to attend, you're ready to push that project 'till the wee hours or fly to Fairbanks on a short-term assignment. Hey, Golda Meir became Israel's prime minister at 70!

When you're returning to work after staying home with kids, don't put yourself down. You haven't "just been a homemaker," you've been fine-tuning your organizational and interpersonal skills. Employers will value you as much as you value yourself. Smaller companies are often willing to "take a chance" on someone who'll be dependable. Work with a temporary agency to get a feel for different environments; they'll often train you in some computer or phone skills. Take some classes or volunteer in a field you're interested in. Rephrase your volunteer work and hobbies in "resume-ese," using an online resume guide. *The Complete Idiot's Guide to the Perfect Resume* shows you how to emphasize strengths and present age and employment gaps in a positive light.

At midlife, we've come to know what's really important in life. So why do all these career change books tell us to be conscious of our "image?" **Like it or not, studies reveal that people decide how smart we are, how much money we make, and what kind of personality we have in the first 8 to 30** seconds, often before we say a word. **What we say and how we say it forms less than half of that first impression. How you dress and how you carry yourself will influence every interaction you have, both in your working and personal lives.** People think women with short, highlighted hair are smarter than women with long, dark curly hair. They think people who exercise are smarter than those who don't. They can't see past the dangly earrings, the wimpy handshake, or the dated clothes into your awesome soul.

You should be changing your eyeglasses and your haircut about every three years. Closed leather pumps, an up-to-date haircut, current eyeglasses, a confident shoulders-back posture, and good eye contact are all hallmarks of a good business look. Check news anchors on TV—they usually have this down. You should look professional, but not rigid or severe. Most dentists will work out a payment plan for the cosmetic work you need to get the teeth looking great; don't skimp on this one and end up with a row of fake-looking Chiclets! Get the right grooming tools to get rid of hair that grows where it didn't used to. Let people feel neutral about your appearance, so they can get to know your opinions and your passions as your relationship unfolds. You can break out the flip-flops and the Hawaiian shirt at the company picnic.

I hear some of you saying, "I've been there and done that with this 'how to get ahead' stuff, and that's how I got into this juggling act in the first place." Seeking more flexibility and self-expression is natural, and many will step off the treadmill, like a lawyer who decided to become a trucker and be closer to his son.

Listen to the little whispers your intuition is sending you from the still, quiet space within. Perhaps you've read and reread that description of the painting class at the community college (whisper). Your girlfriend mentions, out of the blue, she's thinking about taking that very course (loud whisper).

Your daughter compliments your high school painting that hangs in the upstairs hall (shout). The deadline is coming up—surrender to your intuition and sign up already!

If you're dreaming of stepping off—opening an inn, writing a book, becoming a rabbi, operating a dive shop in the Bahamas—be aware that these professions are not an escape. They will require the same professionalism, skills, and time as your current job, seldom provide health insurance, and often require a substantial investment. Sailing the South Seas and hitting the highway sound like fun until you realize that eventually your boat will need repairs and you'll run out of money to buy gas.

Sometimes being in control gets out of control.

The number one deterrent to getting started on your midlife dream is not knowing what it is. The number two problem is perfectionism—that feeling that you can't get started on your dream until you have all your ducks in a row. You act as if everyone will love you and approve of what you're doing if you just do it perfectly.

Lena has acquired every personal trainer certification that exists but hasn't yet trained one person. Why? She doesn't feel "sure of herself." Stephanie has taken every painting course in a 300 mile radius, but hasn't yet set up an easel and had at it, because "people might not like my stuff." Sandy has two unfinished books and an unfinished screenplay in a drawer; if she finishes, she'll have to show someone. **Perfectionism and fear are stealing these women's dreams. You can tell you're doing this when you use the term "Yeah, but..."**—yeah, but I have to wait until after my son graduates or my daughter gets married; yeah, but I don't have a degree/the right degree; yeah, but someone in my life might not like it. Kick your own butt and get rid of the "yeah, buts"!

Your inner perfectionist has you locked in a no-win situation; you fear failing above all, and you can't move ahead without trying and sometimes failing. Your desire to guarantee a successful outcome gets in the way of getting started – you fear failure more than you desire success. The answer, then, is clear—**increase your desire!** Focus on all the positive aspects of achieving your goal until you can move forward without looking over your shoulder and wondering if you're good enough. People admire someone who's willing to strike out and do something badly at first; it gives *them* permission to do the same.

In the story of David and Goliath, David found out that the man who defeated Goliath would marry the princess. He started asking around: "Is she pretty? Does she laugh a lot? How much money does she have? What kind of palace does she live in?" After he had the dream fleshed out, he started flinging those five smooth stones—and you know the rest. **David knew the difference between striving for excellence and striving for perfection;** perfection doesn't exist, but excellence can be built, stone by stone, brick by brick, if you want it badly enough and feed your want with dreams on a regular basis.

Try small changes before you blow up your life.

Resist the pack-up-and-go impulse and try working at an inn or writing your book for two weeks before you chuck everything to get it done. If you plan ahead, you could even cobble together a **sabbatical-size life-change tryout**. Determine what's the slowest time in your industry and plan your vacation plus some weeks of unpaid leave for that time. You must plan ahead for someone to cover your responsibilities and save money to cover those unpaid weeks. Most people are only ninety unpaid days from going broke, so don't be embarrassed if money is an obstacle. Perhaps your search will show you that your current job can be viewed as a cash-generating vehicle for your dreams if you disconnect from the committed mental track you're on. Flirt with your "if only I could" career by moonlighting on weekends, volunteering, or working for cheap; singing in a restaurant, teaching yoga to children, and working in the wardrobe department of a summer theatre can all be called "internships" and "experience."

Several truths stand out:

In this longevity revolution, you're likely to have a long life with varied working situations. The old idea of "retirement" may be obsolete, since few will have the money to do that. In any case, do you really want to play golf and cards for 25 or 30 years? Most people will have at least seven careers in their lifetime, and I see myself building and acquiring skills through my sixties and "sage-ing" and supporting others after that. Care to join me? The alternative stinks.

Those who 'have it all' have found it isn't enough. People are sincerely redefining their definition of success from acquiring things to personal growth and being in control of their lives. If you feel like a chocolate bunny—hollow on the inside—it may be time to scale back your living expenses and get off the "if we just get this, we'll be happy" track. There's always a new opportunity for enthusiastic, committed people.

If it doesn't feel good, don't do it. Or do less of it. Feeling trapped and depressed by your daily routine will have consequences for your health and your relationships. Sometimes you have so much seniority and are so well-compensated for your prison sentence, you feel you can't sign out. But if you don't reexamine, renegotiate, or change *something*, you'll probably shoot yourself in the foot and get booted out anyway. Have you seen the burned-out executive trying desperately to control everyone's actions and holding back progress? Don't be that person. Kick *something* into high gear, and do what it takes to stay engaged and fresh. Start now to develop a life outside your job.

The Checklist

❏ l. Books work best for the in-depth career self-discovery process and fine-tuning your networking skills, but there are sites on the internet you can cruise and get a feel for what's out there. Careerbuilder.com and monster.com have excellent "resources" sections on resumes and interviewing, and you'll find assessments and other tools. Beware of high-priced resume writers and headhunters; read the fine print and know that, in the end, you are responsible for representing yourself. Check idealist.org to look into a job with a nonprofit.

❏ 2. Networking is important in the job hunt and serves another purpose as well—how many people do you know who you can call for help or advice in the middle of the night? The more people you know, the more true friends you'll find who'll step up to the plate at 2 a.m. Trade shows, fundraisers, industry recognition—be there, have a few really good conversations, and incorporate new friends into your life.

❏ 3. In-demand jobs, according to U.S News and World Report 3/3/03: Specialty nurses, medical technicians; librarians with computer skills; school principals, special ed, bilingual, math, and science teachers; slot machine technicians; fitness trainers; network administrator, analysts, internet cops, data-base manager, analyst-developers; loan originators, home-loan sales consultants; financial planners.

❏ **4.** *Entrepreneur* magazine is constantly evaluating business opportunities and helping you do the same; their website has info on start-up costs, raising money, franchises, business plans, e-mail promotion, and using eBay to build your business. *Starting an eBay Business for Dummies* details how to profit online selling everything from jewelry to Bill Clinton bobbleheads.

❏ **5.** Successful real estate broker Barbara Corcoran of The Corcoran Group sells you on selling yourself in *Use What You've Got & Other Business Lessons.* She's got a great way of helping you out of a career slump with chapter titles like "If You Don't Have Big Breasts, Put Ribbons On Your Pigtails."

❏ **6.** If you dream of skipping winter in a warm climate, check out *The Complete Guide to Second Homes for Vacations, Retirement, and Investment.* With tips on hot markets, rental income, negotiating, and financing, author Gary Eldred can have you vacationing now and retiring later in a great investment property.

The Checkup from the Neck Up

❏ I look forward to working with people of intelligence and kindness in creating something that matters.

❏ Looking forward to using the gifts I've been given, I appreciate that all my good and bad experiences will lead to a great future.

❏ At this stage of my life, I have the privilege of exploring what I can be brilliant at, what makes me forget about the passing of time.

❏ I am not "escaping from" but "escaping to" a life I will build, brick by brick, that expresses my best self.

19.

It's My Perimenopause, and I'll Cry If I Want To!

*Your period was 2 weeks late, gushed for 2 weeks, then you didn't
see it for 2 months. You tell your kids "Mommy is having an Evil
Twin day," your mood swings are so bad. Sometimes you feel like
your heart is racing or pounding. You don't care if you ever have
sex again, sometimes sex hurts, you forget names and why you're
in the basement, your breasts feel tender, your pillow is drenched,
and the weight stays or increases no matter what you do.*
Yeah, you're there.

By many accounts, the misery of perimenopause often
peaks at age 47. I was right on schedule, as usual,
experiencing irritability, fatigue, zero interest in sex, urinary
tract infections, and food cravings. **PMS was short for
psychotic mood swings.** For a few days before my period,
nothing anyone said or did seemed right to me. Bloating,
breast tenderness, headaches, lousy sleep, acne—my estrogen
and progesterone were fluctuating, my serotonin was
swinging, and the preperiod blahs got worse through my
forties. The moment I got my light but painful period, the

veil would suddenly be lifted from my entire outlook on life. My family begged me to keep track of my periods and let them know when the three days before my period were coming so they could keep everything "chill". They knew this wasn't the real me and didn't want to hold me responsible for the angry words, the tears, and the slamming doors.

Have you ever heard the expression "I heard my mother coming out of my mouth"? That was me. My mom's angry, sleep-deprived perimenopause was a doozy; at one point, she took off for California and stayed with an aunt after a three-week argument with my father and brother. I remember Dad mumbling to us kids, "Your mother is going through some, uh, changes, so let's just drive to California, pick up Mommy, and have a little vacation." I remember thinking something like the 1968 version of "You go, girl!" (Groovy?) Did her trials and tribulations lead me to expect a difficult transition, even though I'm adopted? Maybe. But at least when the stuff hit the fan, it seemed like a predictable part of the life cycle I could live through.

Like everything else in God's plan, there was a purpose to my psychotic mood swings. For one thing, that's when the idea of writing this book started. As I started to search for answers to why I was feeling bad and what I could do about it, I spoke to other women sharing the same problems. Each woman was so relieved to find that she wasn't going crazy, finding strength and hope in numbers. "Maybe I can help myself, and others too," was the thought that started the files that started the book. It helped me so much to know that these changes were *normal*, and other women were experiencing them at the same time, for the same reasons.

Some journalists have asked "How come there's suddenly this perimenopause thing? Is it just another media invention designed to sell you medication?" This spectrum of symptoms preceding your period that worsens through your late 30's and 40's has probably always been around; two factors account for its increased visibility. Back in the day, just about everything was called "female hysteria" or a "female problem," and what we now call PMS was lumped together with depression, anemia, thyroid deficiency, migraines, allergies, and irritable bowel syndrome—all of which have symptoms related to those of PMS and perimenopause. (Check that thyroid; it's sneaky).

In addition, the high performance lifestyle that women live today make the symptoms seem much more disruptive; environmental toxins and workplace stress can also affect ovarian function. Your jam-packed itinerary may leave little time for the extra naps, exercise, frequent small meals, and anti-stress activities like massage and meditation that would help you feel better. Okay, I hear you laughing at that prescription! But seriously, if the issue is performing at work and serving others, how will you do that if *you're* a frazzled mess? In their 40's and 50's, women who take care of themselves with exercise, sleep, sunshine, less caffeine, healthy (cut the white bread and sugar) eating and annual checkups pull ahead of the pack. Their chain-smoking, coffee-guzzling, live-on-the-edge sisters start to look just plain *old*, and *feel* even worse.

Beyond self-care, your first line of defense is consistently taking your multi with 400 mg Vitamin E and good old calcium with magnesium. In a recent study, being really consistent with 1,200 mg/day of calcium for three full cycles cut symptoms *in half* for women suffering from water retention, food cravings, lower-back pain, and low mood. Dr. Herbert Benson's famous *Relaxation Response*

(Chapter 33) can help you conquer hot flashes and anxiety. Many women also find relief with Thermacare heat pads, bright-light therapy, massage, and herbals like vitex (see Chapter 7). A good massage therapist would be willing to negotiate an inexpensive rate for two 30-minute massages during the premenstrual week, particularly if it's during her off-peak hours. If you find that after three months of calcium, less caffeine, and more sleep you need more help, the next step is oral contraceptives (OCs), but start with a *certain kind* of OC. My gyno prescribed Loestrin for my PMS symptoms, and I felt so bad I threw them out after six weeks. I felt as if I was wading through quicksand on a daily basis, both physically and mentally.

For non-smoking women, OCs (birth control pills) are a midlife bonanza! Where else can you get 1) contraception 2) *decreased* risk of endometrial and ovarian cancers, fibrocystic breasts, and uterine fibroids 3) regulation of heavy and irregular periods 4) results against PMS, endometriosis, menstrual migraines, acne, and ovarian cysts 5) and prevent bone loss? Check out this scenario: you breeze through your late thirties and forties taking the right kind of birth control pills; at 51, you find your FSH level is high and go on bioidentical low-dose hormones to waltz happily through the menopausal transition. Are you *cool*, or what?

But don't start out with a prescription for *low-estrogen* OCs like Alesse, Mircette, LoOvral, Loestrin, and Ortho-Novum; these tend to aggravate mood swings and weight gain, not help them. Instead, advises *Screaming to be Heard* author Dr. Elizabeth Lee Vliet, the birth control pills "using less than 1 mg of norethindrone (or equivalent) with 30 to 35 mcg of ethinyl estradiol are the ones I have found less likely to over stimulate your appetite and contribute to weight gain.

Examples of these are Ovcon 35, Modicon, Yasmin, Diane 35 in Canada, and Ortho-Cyclen." Spot bleeding usually goes away after a few months. If none of these work for you after a while, see if the Ortho Evra Patch or (vaginal) Nuvaring have a better metabolic effect for you, or swing the other way to the Loestrin 1/20-type pill. A good discussion of these different OCs is at wdxcyber.com.

Seasonale is a new OC taken for 84 days in a row, followed by a week of placebos. For women with horrible cramps, acne, mood swings, and asthma and migraines that get worse premenstrually, the idea of having only four periods a year is very attractive. Doctors have been prescribing other OC's off-label to be used this way for years. The daily progestin keeps the uterine lining from building up, so the need to bleed each month is decreased. Is it safe? Supposedly, the estrogen/progestin content and overall hormone exposure is lower, and the system duplicates the fact that back in the day, women had fewer periods because they were always pregnant. (Ain't it great to be a 21st Century Girl?!) If your current OC is working well, work with your doctor to try the period-skipping routine by just throwing away the placebo pills, starting with the next pack, and stopping for four days to bleed about every three months. Don't forget; write it in your calendar or put a tickler on your computer.

Staying on the right OC on a continuous regimen through your 40's solves the **heavy bleeding** for many women, including those with endometriosis and fibroids. You can often take a wait-and-see attitude with birth control pills, since symptoms are controlled; pelvic pain is less frequent and later, menopause will cause fibroids to shrink. A very low dose (5-10 mg) of mifepristone taken daily for six months, shrinks fibroids by half and relieves heavy periods and lower back pain.

Some women have been empowered to control their pain with the right diet, as in *Endometriosis: A Key to Healing Through Nutrition* or *Healing Fibroids*. Laparoscopic surgery (*not* hysterectomy) by a skilled specialist both diagnoses and treats endometriosis, as she can laser off lesions and release adhesions while confirming the diagnosis. A D&C or an endometrial ablation—including Uterine Balloon Therapy or the Hydro Therm Ablator—are other options that have calmed the pelvic storm for many women. Check *all* your options; your physician tends to recommend the procedure *they're* trained in, because that's what they're most familiar with.

Think twice before becoming a hyster-sister!

Though as many as 50% of US women have **fibroids**, most will not cause symptoms. But for those who have bleeding, cramping, and backache; those with fibroids so large, you're dressing to disguise it; and if you're more than six years away from menopause, you may want to consider removing the fibroids with myomectomy or uterine artery embolization. Other great therapies are on the horizon; the team at Boston Brigham and Women's Hospital recently used an ultrasound beam to kill fibroid tissue, guided by an MRI.

The last resort for fibroid complications or any pelvic problem during perimenopause is hysterectomy. The surgery doesn't always fix your problems, and sometimes adds *more* complications to the problems you already have. Don't give up your uterus, cervix, and ovaries without considering all the options! They all serve your body throughout your life in ways we don't fully understand. The uterus and cervix are part of your orgasmic response, and hysterectomy can cause genital nerve damage, pain during intercourse, and wacky hormones. When a doctor suggests you "take it all out, you don't need them, you're done having children," ask if men should have *their* sexual organs removed when they don't want to conceive. If you have sexual side effects from a hysterectomy, don't let anyone tell you it's "all in your head."

No, you should not have a hysterectomy because your fibroid *could* get bigger or it *could* be cancerous or it *could* be hiding an ovary with a problem. Explore your options thoroughly with a second opinion, reading books like *Your Guide to Hysterectomy, Ovary Removal, and Hormone Replacement* and *The Woman's Guide to Hysterectomy*, and checking out the Hyster Sisters and nohysterectomy.com websites. It makes all the difference if you know all your choices and finally *choose* to have a hysterectomy. It does help women with cancer and some women with heavy bleeding, prolapsed uterus, and pelvic pain, and — when combined with bioidentical hormone therapy to balance the sudden change—can smooth the midlife transition.

Menstrual migraines can be much worse during perimenopause. Start taking ibuprofen or other pain relievers two days before your regular period, or at the first sign of headache if your periods are irregular. Some have success with daily use of 150 mg of CoQ10 or the herb feverfew, or with a regimen of 400 mg of riboflavin (B2) and magnesium. Don't wait until the migraine is intense. Jump into bed and give yourself a "personal day" at the first pre-headache flash of light in your vision. A new migraine med called Frova seems to work better for menstrual migraines because they stay in the bloodstream longer than other triptans. Botox injections may stop nerves from sending pain signals to the brain. Exercise, yoga, consistent eating and sleeping schedules, acupuncture and biofeedback help migraines, along with avoiding trigger foods like the 4 c's—cheese, chocolate, caffeine, and citrus.

Red wine, aspartame, and MSG can also promote migraines.

Migraine sufferers might consider doing the period-skipping routine with their OC's (see above), or they can try using a low-dose estrogen patch or pill during the week off the regular OCs. The drop in estrogen before your period causes migraines, so you can "...bump up your estrogen levels by taking 1 mg or lower of estrogen (17 beta-estradiol) twice a day starting 2 or 3 days prior to your period and continuing for 2 or 3 days into your period. For less predictable migraines, a dissolvable form of estrogen placed under the tongue can be used as needed," according to Dr. Mary Jane Minkin in her excellent column in *Prevention* magazine. Ask your pharmacist or check the pharmacies listed in Chapter 21 about a very low dose of sublingual estrogen.

For bloating, the only diuretic that really pulls the plug on PMS water-logging is Spironolactone (Aldactone). 100 mg daily, taken for the 14 days before your period, reduces abdominal bloating and may improve other symptoms as well. I swore my brain was as bloated as my belly, and research seems to uphold that. Thiazide diuretics won't have the same effect, and you may not need a diuretic if you find an OC that works for you.

Symptom Relief with SSRI's

If you still have bad symptoms after all these approaches, it's time to look at the mood meds, SSRI's like Prozac. Experiment with Prozac, Zoloft, Paxil, Luvox, and Celexa for 10 to 14 days before your period; each has a slightly different "feel" so it may take a while to get the right one. Many women have good PMS mood results with a premenstrual dose of Prozac as low as 2 mg, and also see improvements in other symptoms. SSRI antidepressants work on the drop in the brain chemical serotonin that precedes your period.

Serafem, marketed as "Prozac for PMS," is just high-priced Prozac, since the original happy pill has gone off patent. Cymbalta is a new antidepressant that targets two brain chemicals and may work for a broader spectrum of depressed patients.

The makers of both Paxil and Effexor have published studies showing **significant hot flash relief** for women taking low doses of their drugs. To counteract the lack of desire and orgasm that are typical side effects of SSRI's, some have success using a low dose of Wellbutrin XR, a MAOI type of antidepressant, two hours before sex. You could also consider substituting Wellbutrin XR for the SSRI's, and see how that feels. EmSam is a new MAOI patch that works more quickly than oral drugs. Don't stop these drugs abruptly, taper off—they can have **nasty withdrawal symptoms**.

Many other drugs affect antidepressants, causing a rare but serious reaction called "serotonin syndrome." Parkinson's drugs, migraine drugs like Imitrex, OTC drugs for colds like dextromethorphan, St. John's Wort, Meridia, Dexedrine, and Tegretol are among these interactors. These mirth medications are no joke—*please* have a complete checkup with blood work testing your thyroid and ovarian hormones before you mess with your brain chemistry.

The Checklist

❏ I. Don't take St. John's Wort with your oral contraceptive; it may decrease the contraceptive effectiveness of the OC by as much as 50% and you could get pregnant. Tell your doctor about any supplements you're taking before *any* drug is prescribed. Soy foods and some herbs, for example, can aggravate endometriosis.

❏ **2.** If you still need birth control but absolutely cannot stand any kind of hormones, condoms are the obvious choice. But there's a new kid on the block who moved away and came back to the neighborhood—the Today Sponge. Though it's currently available on Canada's birthcontrol.com, you can check progress on U.S. availability on Todaysponge.com. Immortalized on *Seinfeld* as Elaine's favorite birth control, the sponge is not messy, can be bought without a prescription, and can be inserted well in advance of having sex.

❏ **3.** A new sterilization technique will be an alternative to the anesthesia and recovery period of tubal ligation. The quick-recovery Essure technique uses a catheter to place a device that blocks the Fallopian tube. Tissue grows around the device, and it becomes a permanent implant preventing pregnancy.

❏ **4.** Nutrition specialist Ann Louise Gittleman offers a natural do-it-yourself kit for perimenopause in her book, *Before the Change*. **Ann Louise's All-Star Peri Zappers:** Flaxseed Oil, Evening Primrose Oil (GLA), Multivitamin and Magnesium, Zinc, Natural Progesterone Cream, Exercise, Destressing Stress, Adrenal Refresher, Soy Phytoestrogens, Natural Hormone Therapy. Her endorsements of adrenal glandulars, estriol, and tri-estrogen are controversial, but many benefit from her program.

❏ **5.** I hate to cast doubt on the love affair, but here it is: soy and other phytoestrogens like vitex may compete at receptor sites with estradiol, the energy hormone, giving you even less energy, interfering with ovulation, thyroid, and bone-building, and causing possible sleeplessness, according to Dr. Vliet in *It's My Ovaries, Stupid!* "I heard soy was good" is not enough of a reason to load up without monitoring your responses. She prescribes DHEA but advises not to use over-the-counter DHEA, as current studies show adverse effects on declining estradiol.

❑ **6.** How do you know when to switch from low-dose birth control pills to bioidentical hormone replacement? On days 5, 6, or 7 of the placebo-pill week, have the FSH level of your blood tested. If it's over 20 mIU/ml, it may be time to switch to the even lower doses of estradiol and progesterone in hormone replacement. Age 51 is the average, but smoking, a tubal ligation, medications, family trends and many other factors can cause menopause to come earlier or later.

❑ **7.** Heavy menstrual bleeding can also be caused by Von Willibrands (a blood clotting disorder, often with nosebleeds and bruising), polyps, and adenomyosis (an endometrial problem).

The Checkup from the Neck Up

❑ When I feel my body is out of control, I remember my attitude is under *my* control.

❑ My body is changing to accommodate the growth of my wisdom, my experience, and my growing confidence.

❑ I listen to what my body is telling me about my past, my present, and my future.

❑ I acknowledge that my midlife transformation is part of the process that will reveal the direction of the rest of my life.

20.

Get It While You're Hot
There is an alternative to the
dangerous HRT you've heard about.

*"More women know their options and know that they can change
their regimens if they're not working. They have access to a wealth
of new information about menopausal physiology and medicine.
Above all, their HRT options have increased dramatically just over
the last five years. Today the question 'Do I need or want HRT?'
is, in fact, a series of questions, including 'What kind?'
'What strength?' 'In what combination?" For what reason?'
'For how long' and 'At what risk?'*
—Christiane Northrup M.D., The Wisdom of Menopause.

You may be one of those women who sails through
perimenopause and menopause without symptoms—and that's
great! Healthy as could be, with the bone density and annual
checkup results to prove it! You can skip this chapter, or go
ahead and read it so you're informed enough to help friends, or
notice changes in yourself you may not have attributed to
hormone levels. From the age of 42 on, I've had every
hormone imbalance symptom there is, and may have invented

some new ones! Yet, I would never consider taking what most people think of as "hormones," the standard 0.0625 mg dose of conjugated equine estrogen (see the 4 P's below) that was widely prescribed.

I've noticed three ways women experience menopause. The lucky ones appear puzzled by a discussion of symptoms. Their usual comment is, "I just stopped having periods, and that was that." Another group gets the mood swings, tougher PMS, headaches, and hot flashes, but they hop on the internet, sleep more, try some herbals, whole grains, and yoga, and go from being the "Den Mother to the Zen Mother" without many problems. A healthy lifestyle and the suggestions in Chapter 6 are all they need to fast- forward to post-menopausal zest.

The final 30% are Les Menopause Miserables: they only go to restaurants with great air conditioning, since they always carry their own tropical weather. They have heart palpitations, anxiety attacks, rage, rogue chin whiskers, giant fibroids, and non-stick memories. The dryness of their vaginas is only exceeded by their lack of sexual desire; and their leakage of urine and gas may occasionally be surpassed by the avalanche of their very heavy periods. They're not snack-snarfing, TV-watching slackers—they do some decent self-care. "I'm *already* exercising and eating right, I'm *doing* all that," they say, "I just want to feel like my self again!" Maybe they're high-powered professionals who are constantly in the public eye and have to perform at a high level despite tough symptoms. Les Menopause Miserables are the ones who should consider at least a few years of bioidentical hormone replacement before they punch out of the menopausal time clock.

If you've had a lot of mind and body changes like me, you may be taking fistfuls of vitamins and herbals; antibiotics for frequent urinary infections; Prozac, Effexor, or Paxil for depression; the latest miracle supplement for weight loss; and a shelf full of medications for sleep, cholesterol, and blood pressure problems. **This is like chasing papers in the wind instead of putting your foot on the stack! Did it ever occur to you that these changes started as you got older, and they might have a common cause? Are you attacking the symptoms instead of looking at the root of the problem—hormone changes?**

In her book, *Women, Weight, and Hormones*, Dr. Elizabeth Lee Vliet applies the vast knowledge of her women-centered medical practice and her previous book, *Screaming to be Heard*, to the problem of weight gain. Dr. Vliet contends that you should consider balancing your hormones, particularly rapidly declining estradiol, in dealing with weight gain and other bothersome midlife symptoms. She urges you to seek reliable serum (blood) testing and bioidentical hormone solutions, **not** to attribute all your symptoms to "stress" (the new millennium's version of "hysteria"), and she looks at the whole woman, not just the weight problem:

"Estradiol contributes to improved insulin response, enhanced energy and mood, as well as clarity of thinking, sharper memory, ability to concentrate, normal blood pressure, optimal bone density, better quality of sleep, a better sex drive, and a healthy, active metabolic rate. Declining estradiol during midlife also contributes to a decrease in serotonin production. Loss of optimal serotonin, in turn, causes depression, increased irritability, increased anxiety, increased pain sensitivity, eating disorders, increased obsessive-compulsive thinking, and increased disruption of normal sleep rhythms. Each of these effects can make your metabolism more sluggish, so the cumulative result of losing your optimal estradiol is that it is now harder for you to lose excess fat."

Other problems that Dr. Vliet shows may be linked to midlife hormone changes are Alzheimer's, macular degeneration, sleep apnea, alcoholism complications, gallstones, gastro esophageal reflux disease (GERD), dry and sagging skin, dry eyes (and contact lens problems), thinning hair and hair loss, and sinus problems. I still marvel at the difference in my brain when I've forgotten to change my patch; thinking is like walking at the bottom of the ocean. Then I change it, and have a "This is your dead brain; this is your blossoming brain on estradiol" moment. In addition to the memory, mood, sleep, concentration, and sex drive benefits, I noticed a lot less dental bleeding and gum recession when I started the estradiol patch. **Think about the cost of the doctor visits, tests, treatments, and medications for all these conditions, and no one tests hormone levels or attempts hormone balance to see if they are related!** Du-uh!

The 4 P's—the bad ones you've heard about!

The widely used hormone replacement regimen you've heard about in the Women's Health Initiative—the study that was halted in 2002 when the heart disease and breast cancer risks outweighed the drug's benefits—is represented by the four P's – Premarin, Provera, Prempro, and PremPhase. **When someone recommends bioidentical hormones, they are <u>NOT</u> recommending these products!** Premarin, a conjugated estrogenic product made from pregnant mare's urine, combined with Provera, a synthetic form of progesterone called a progestin, has been the most-prescribed regimen for menopausal symptoms since the 1950's. It was convenient for doctors to prescribe this one-size-fits-all regimen, sometimes called "the longest experiment ever performed on women." Prempro, the specific hormone combination used in the Women's Health Initiative, is Premarin plus a progestin in the same daily pill, while PremPhase adds the progestin for two weeks of the month. In 2003, analysis of the WHI data also found that older women who took Prempro for long periods of time doubled their risk of developing Alzheimer's and other cognitive problems, and had a higher risk of breast cancer, heart attacks, and strokes.

In her book *Is It Hot In Here Or Is It Me?*, author Gayle Sand humorously expresses the feelings many of us have about hormones made from pregnant mare's urine:

"I am a free-range person. I don't eat anything that has chemicals, additives, or preservatives. I eat foods that have a shelf-life, not a half-life. When the ingredients listed on the side of a package sound like they should be in a hand grenade, I don't buy the product. If something's pickled, smoked, or cured I won't touch it. In my opinion, if it's cured it had to be sick to begin with. I refuse to turn my body into a chemical dumping ground filled with nitrites, pesticides, dyes, waxes, and fumigants. If it's artificial, imitation, or synthetic I won't go near it. I am a natural person. Menopause is a natural process. It is not natural to put hormones made from the urine of a horse in my system. Any claims to the contrary, as far as I'm concerned, are pure horse manure."

The side effects commonly associated with HRT—irritability, depression, and loss of desire—are often attributed to the synthetic progestins (different from progesterone) in these products. A friend on Prempro said to me, "Okay, I'm sleeping better, but everything my husband does irritates me. Not to mention the three B's – bloating, breast tenderness, and unpredictable bleeding." Many women quit the "P" regimens after a few months. Women know that the less progestin they take, the better they feel. Why not avoid the synthetic stuff altogether, and look at other products that replace what's missing, in formulas identical to the ones your body produces?

The common wisdom - from sources like magazines, health web sites, and your doctor—*used* to state that Premarin, Provera, Prempro, and PremPhase protected against heart disease and osteoporosis and relieved menopausal symptoms. "This is the standard that's been tested, this is the one we know the most about," they would say.

Studies in the 80's and early 90's came out to support the benefits of this one-size-fits-all regimen for those conditions, as well as relief from depression, midlife sexual changes, and even Alzheimer's disease. There were two problems with these studies:

1. some of them were supported by the company that makes Premarin, and

2. for the most part, they did not use any other form of hormone replacement to compare results.

It's not surprising, then, that the hormonal house of cards fell down in the summer of 2002, when the Women's Health Initiative halted the trial using Prempro when researchers found *more* heart attacks, strokes, blood clots, and breast cancer in women on the drug. In August of 2003, the Million Woman study at Britain's Cancer Research UK showed much higher breast cancer rates among participants using a combined regimen similar to the one used in the WHI trial. Doctors' and patients' attitudes turned on a dime, and millions of women went cold turkey, determined to grin and bear symptoms and give up all forms of hormone replacement forever. It's no mystery why women are afraid—the words "hormone," "cancer," and "heart disease" seem linked in the media.

In her best-selling book, **The Wisdom of Menopause**, Dr. Christiane Northrup addresses the most common risk factors for hormone replacement. Read carefully as this wise and compassionate doctor speaks to your most common fear in these paragraphs:

"Factor 7: You are at increased risk for breast, uterine, ovarian, or bowel cancer. A positive personal or family history for one or more of these hormone-related cancers makes the hormone replacement decision very anxiety-provoking for many women. Here are the facts: Recent research has suggested that the dose and formulation of HRT are important factors in the cancer issue. Though all types of estrogen at high enough doses over a long period of time can potentially stimulate breast cancer growth, I feel that Premarin, because of its association with DNA damage and because it has a stronger biological effect than bioidentical estrogens, may be more carcinogenic than bioidentical estrogens. In other words, the increased risk of breast and uterine cancer shown by past studies may have been related to estrogenic overdose or the wrong kind of estrogen, rather than estrogen per se. If estrogen is taken in a way that more closely mimics the way it is produced in the body—in physiological doses calibrated to the body's needs, in bioidentical formulation, and partnered with bioidentical, not synthetic, progesterone—it begins to lose its sinister profile."

Drs Northrup and Vliet address the hormone question from every possible medical/holistic/emotional angle in their books. It's a complex question.

It's your life; look into it!

Please don't think you know all about hormones because of a few sound bites you heard on TV! Stop flapping your lips with "I heard it causes cancer" when you don't even know what "it" is. Stop believing people who tell you your symptoms are just stress. Stop swallowing drug company hype or media hysteria, and give the question a serious look. Stop taking medications for each symptom—depression, migraines, urinary infections, memory loss—without answering the hormone question. Then decide what *you* want to do to feel better.

Yes, there's a lot of controversy and a lack of good studies, but that's true in every area of women's health. An oversimplified blip of news about cancer gets everyone's attention, while a complicated story about glowing health gets no one's. Cancer is a disease of aging. Hormones are a natural part of your body. Young women with the highest hormone levels have the lowest cancer levels; estrogen replacement *reduces* colon cancer and osteoporosis; and birth control pills *reduce* your risk of endometrial and ovarian cancer. Back in Bible days, you had your first baby at 12, and by the time you were 40 you were probably dead. We can't know the long-term consequences of many things, because "long-term" is a relatively new concept. You didn't *need* to create this high-demand new second life for yourself, and hormones were the least of your worries.

Don't think of hormone replacement as a lifelong choice!

For some reason, women have this misconception that they'll go to their graves taking hormones once they start. Fuggettaboudit! Since the Women's Health Initiative, the thinking is—use the lowest dose of bioidentical hormones that relieves your symptoms for six months, a year, three years, and then reevaluate. You can use them for a year, and decide every year on your birthday whether to continue or not. It's up to you!

With our longer life expectancy, there's a natural desire to improve the quality of all those extra years. We all know that a healthy diet, exercise, and appropriate check-ups and testing are our first line of defense, but bioidentical hormone replacement can be an important part of that plan. There are women who need to give some careful thought to the type and route of delivery if they want to take hormones. They include women who have:

- a history of uterine, endometrial or breast cancer or two first-degree relatives with these cancers
  - a strong family history of cancer
  - existing heart disease and stroke
  - migraines
  - benign fibroids
  - endometriosis

Some women should only consider using estradiol in the form of the transdermal patch, which allows the hormone to initially bypass the liver and reduces the amount of estrone delivered to the body. The patch may be the safest form of estrogen to use (See Dr. Vliet's list in *The Checklist*). Use of the estrogen patch or estrogen vaginal cream over oral forms should especially be considered over other forms by those who have:

- hypertension
- clotting and circulation problems such as varicose veins
- diabetes
- liver disease
- gallbladder disease
- migraines

All this information can be very intimidating at first, but don't decide by listening to random news reports and your friends. Read some books; surf some credible sources on the Internet or ask a friend to print some articles for you. I know that sometimes your goal is just to make it through the day, but over several months you can pick up a lot of information if you write it in your calendar, put a book on your bedside, and nibble away at your quest.

The Checklist

• Patches keep blood levels of estradiol fairly steady, similar to the hormone production by the ovary (helpful for women with blood pressure or "hormonal" headache problems).

• Estradiol by patch gives better improvement in glucose control and insulin sensitivity than oral estrogens.

• Patches do not lead to further elevation of estrone (as seen with oral forms) since the estradiol bypasses the liver first pass.

• Estradiol in a patch is less likely to be affected by other medications, since the estradiol is not metabolized first in the liver.

• Transdermal delivery of estradiol does not elevate triglycerides as occurs in some women taking oral estrogens.

• Estradiol by patch is less likely to cause gallstones.

• Patches maintain benefits of estradiol on HDL to LDL cholesterol even though this form of estradiol delivery doesn't raise HDL as rapidly or quite as high as oral estrogens. *List from **Women, Weight, and Hormones**, by* Elizabeth Lee Vliet,M.D.

21.

Natural Hormones
Stop Denying and Start Flying

"Postmenopause estrogen therapy (ET) dramatically reduces risk of heart disease and osteoporosis, yet less than 15% of postmenopausal women take estrogen, in part because of an exaggerated fear of breast cancer in media reports…In our practice, we encounter daily examples of…health plans that would rather pay $100-200 every month for Prozac or Zoloft or Celexa, but say 'it's too expensive' to check hormone levels and find out that what a woman may need could be thyroid or ovary hormone options that might cost $20 a month."
—**Elizabeth Lee Vliet, M.D.**, Screaming to Be Heard

Luckily for the Midlife Mamas of today, the truth is coming out about better ways to do hormone replacement. "The naturals"—plant-based hormones identical to the ones your body produces—have been around for many years. In Europe, many different forms of native human estradiol, progesterone, and testosterone are routinely prescribed, and doctors are aware of the nuances of different gels, patches, creams, and pills. "Old school" doctors here in America have still been clunking along, prescribing the "cookbook" approach with Premarin, Provera, and Prempro horse-derived estrogen pills. Now that recent studies have made women terrified of all estrogens, the docs are ready to throw the baby out with the bath water, confusing these "P" regimens with more natural bioidentical hormones.

An important hormone described in the previous chapter is estradiol, the strongest of the three types of estrogen your body makes, and the one we're usually referring to when we talk about "estrogen." In very, very simplified terms, estrogen is the energy-and-mental-focus hormone, and progesterone calms things down and helps you sleep, so you take it before bed. Estrace and Gynodiol tablets, Estragel in Canada, and Vivelle DOT, Fempatch, Estraderm, and Climara patches are some of the brand names delivering estradiol, and women with a uterus must combine them with bioidentical progesterone products to protect the endometrium. The Vivelle DOT estradiol patch looks like a piece of clear tape about the size of a postage stamp, and you can exercise, shower, and swim without giving it a second thought. Check out their web site at vivelledot.com. The Climara patch's claim to fame is its once-a-week change regimen (berlex.com). **Blood tests reveal the perfect dose for you, but a typical starting low-dose regimen might be:**

1. Vivelle DOT .0375 patch, changed twice a week, with Prometrium 200 mg for 12 days of the month

2. or the patch plus Prochieve vaginal gel 4% every other night for 12 nights of the month.

3. Estrace tablets 0.5 daily with Prometrium 200 mg for 12 days of the month.

Many women heard about the naturals for the first time on *Oprah*, when the great daytime diva was searching for the reason for her perimenopause-induced heart palpitations. One of the bioidentical naturals mentioned on the show is progesterone, available in many forms, including pills, creams, and gels. 1995's PEPI study found that bioidentical progesterone had fewer side effects and better cardiovascular effects than synthetic progestins like the one in Prempro. Two of the "positive P" brand names you can find are Prometrium, a prescription-only pill with oral micronized natural progesterone, and ProGest, an over-the-counter progesterone cream. Prochieve vaginal gel 4% is another prescription form of bioidentical progesterone, used in menopause with an estradiol patch or pill to deliver progesterone vaginally, directly to the uterus.

Blood, saliva, or urine testing can determine your need for these and other hormones, though blood tests are still the most reliable way to go. I asked my internist to include ovarian hormone testing in my annual physical's blood work, and he told me they don't recommend that because "hormones vary." I replied that "Cholesterol varies too, and that's a pretty common test, so how about if we give it a try?" That made sense to him, and the results, shared with my gynecologist, showed that it was time to kick my estrogen patch up a notch. You must find a doctor who will either know about these things or be willing to read the carefully selected research you find about it. Respect the doctor's professionalism, and she will respect your intelligence.

My girlfriend's doctor gave her the old saw about "absorption from the patch varies and it doesn't prevent osteoporosis like the oral forms." Get with the program, doc! Absorption is actually more like your body's own system (See Dr. Vliet's list in previous chapter), and bone-retaining benefits take a few months to kick in. When you are further down the road, you may want to avoid menstrual-type bleeding by taking a continuous regimen of 1.0 Estrace or 0.1 Vivelle DOT with 100 mg Prometrium each night. Prescription Activella tablets work well for some women who want a combined pill and don't want monthly bleeding, though they do have a low dose of synthetic progestin with the bioidentical estradiol. Users of the new Femring in a Hyster Sisters chat room were enthusiastic about the convenience of changing it every 3 months, but the vaginal ring contains estradiol acetate, not the bioidentical form. Migraine sufferers should try the patch form of estradiol with natural micronized progesterone and consider adding a low dose of testosterone. If you're taking oral estradiol, dividing your Estrace into morning and evening doses can also help avoid headaches.

For symptoms starting in perimenopause, when you're still menstruating and could get pregnant, a low progestin birth control pill is probably your best choice (see chapter 19). I started the Vivelle patch/progesterone regimen in my late forties for my perimenopause symptoms because I had a tubal ligation at 35, and didn't need the higher-dose birth control pills for contraception. Some of the other estradiol patch brands were larger and kept falling off, so I became an expert at covering them up with extra band-aids to keep them on (not very attractive). But the Vivelle DOT just hung in there, helping me feel like myself again in so many ways. **The beauty of Vivelle, Climara, Estrace, Prometrium, Prochieve, and other brand-name bioidenticals is that you can buy them through any pharmacy, your doctor has probably heard of them, and they are FDA-approved and standardized, so they'll likely be covered through your insurance.**

Estriol cream, Vagifem vaginal tablets, Estrace cream, and the Estring vaginal ring deliver localized estradiol when **vaginal dryness or urinary tract problems** are the focus. "Vaginal atrophy" is the medical term for a thin, inflamed vaginal lining caused by lack of estrogen. (Funny, that doesn't seem like much of "A Trophy".) The Estring is probably the lowest consistent source of estrogen available, and can be considered by women who are contraindicated for estrogen use, like those who've had breast cancer. Compounded estriol vaginal cream 0.5 mg is another option for vaginal dryness, especially for women who don't want to use estradiol but absolutely can't tolerate another UTI or painful intercourse. I had a reaction to something in the Estrace cream my urologist recommended, but tolerated the Vagifem tablets (no propylene glycol) really well. If you only use moisture replacements like Astroglide or silk-E, you're treating the symptoms but not the source of the problem, which is hormone changes that will worsen.

The "Mercedes" of hormone regimens is to have a knowledgeable doctor measure your hormones and prescribe a custom, dye-and-preservative-free version to be made up by a compounding pharmacist. Many doctors are reluctant to prescribe these because they're worried about consistency and reliability and just aren't knowledgeable about it. All kinds of bioidentical formulations are available—in pills, creams, gels, and tablets you melt under your tongue—and you may have to work through a few regimens before you feel completely comfortable. I had the hardest time finding a hormone-smart doctor, so I worked it backwards; I called a pharmacist listed in the yellow pages as a compounding pharmacist, and asked him what doctors were sending him prescriptions for bioidentical hormones. Voila!

The pharmacists listed in *The Checklist* at the end of this chapter: have info and complete bioidentical-testing-and-hormone programs on their websites; may mail you a list of doctors who've used them; and can also talk directly with your current doctor. Print out some info that you believe describes you from these sites, from Dr's Vliet, Northrup, and Corio's books, and from this book, and get them to your doctor a week or two *before* you meet with her. Shoving it in her face at the appointment gives her no chance to check into whether she should order testing or write you a prescription.

How about that energetic, sexy hormone testosterone, the one we associate with Monday night football? The big T is definitely the go-to hormone when the problem is lack of desire and sexual interest, and we'll take a hard look in Chapter 14. A testosterone patch for women called Intrinsa is in the pipeline, but meanwhile we must take a passion pill, melt a tab under the tongue, or rub on a cream.

Hormone Controversies

Estrogen or progesterone? Blood tests, saliva tests, or "see how you feel on this"? Safe or not? Testosterone or DHEA? Though many of the physicians writing about hormones are united in their opposition to Premarin and the other animal-derived and synthetic P's, they differ on other aspects of hormone replacement. Drs. John R. Lee and Jesse Hanley argue that *too much* estrogen or "estrogen dominance" is characteristic of peri- and menopause and advocate small physiologic doses of natural progesterone for most midlife symptoms in their books, *What Your Doctor May Not Tell You about Menopause* and *What Your Doctor May Not Tell You about Premenopause*. Studies on USP progesterone cream benefits go both ways, but wild yam creams have been shown to have no effect.

Marla Ahlgrimm, founder of the women-centered Madison Pharmacy, and John M. Kells, CEO of Aeron LifeCycles Clinical Laboratory, advocate saliva testing of hormone levels in their book *The HRT Solution*. They argue that less-expensive saliva testing can be done more often to achieve effective, safe levels faster, and that this testing picks up subtle levels of hormones other tests miss. Reputable studies published in the last three years dispute this.

Is bioidentical hormone replacement absolutely safe? No, we can't say that about any medication, really. The ongoing Women's Health Initiative should tell us more, but in the meantime, two groups of women should definitely consider it— women recovering from the "instant menopause" of hysterectomy and those with symptoms that interfere with their high-demand life. Keep it low-dose and limited-time if you have risk factors and fears about cancer.

The Checklist

❏ **I.** Just putting "bioidentical hormones" or "compounding pharmacies" in your search engine will give you some idea of the widespread interest in natural hormones. There are some phonies out there hawking junky creams and supplements though, so be careful. Power-surge.com is an interesting web site.

❏ **2.** To find a compounding pharmacist near you, put your zip code in the International Association of Compounding Pharmacist's site, iacprx.org. Some of these guys may be in the "saliva kit testing" business; a knowledgeable pharmacist is a great ally, but is not your physician.

❏ **3.** Belmar Pharmacy 800-525-9473, belmarpharmacy.com
• College Pharmacy – collegepharmacy.com
• Madison Pharmacy 800-558-7046, womenshealth.com
• Natural Woman Institute 888-489-6626, naturalwoman.org
• Spence Pharmacy 800-209-7364
• College Pharmacy has a good discussion of gels,

sublingual tabs, pellet implants, suppositories, and other delivery methods of bioidentical hormone replacement. Some of these sites have lists of doctors who regularly prescribe bioidentical hormones and helpful articles about women's' health issues.

❑ **4.** *Screaming to be Heard*, 2nd edition, Elizabeth Lee Vliet M.D., is the "bible" of books about midlife physical changes and hormones. It's large and intimidating-looking, but well worth the effort. Buy it, borrow it, whatever you need to do—but you will know more than your doctor when you read what this caring, passionate doctor has to say! Also read her take on the WHI study and other hormone headlines on her web site, herplace.com.

22.

Go With the Flow
Keep that urinary tract flowing and glowing!

Midlife is when:
* *you go to the doctor and realize you now have to pay someone to look at you naked.*
* *your memory really starts to go and the only thing you still retain is water.*
* *you no longer have upper arms; you have wingspans.*
* *hair growth on your legs slows down so you can spend time on your new mustache and chin hairs.*

You can't make it through an aerobics class without going to the bathroom. When you sneeze or laugh unexpectedly, you wet yourself. Long movies are a problem, and a full night's sleep is a thing of the past. You have a funny pressure down there, or a not-so-funny burning sensation. After making love, you often get the burning or the itching or both. Sometimes when you stand up after urinating, you sit right back down and go again. You have a long history of urinary tract infections, and lately it seems as if antibiotics aren't working. When you gotta go, you gotta go *now*! What's going on here?

Starting around age 35, several factors combine to cause

urinary problems. **Nerve damage** from childbirth, surgery, or smoking can throw things out of alignment. **Loss of estrogen** causes urethral tissues to thin, causing recurrent bladder infections (cystitis), vaginal infections, and incontinence. Antidepressants, statins, antihistamines, heart and heartburn drugs, and many other medications aggravate the bladder and urinary tract. In addition, you may have forgotten those Kegel exercises you learned in childbirth class, and your **pelvic floor muscles have gotten weaker.**

I am the poster girl for this set of symptoms, starting at age 9 with my first urinary tract infection (clue—I also started my period at 9). The hormonal fluctuations right before your period often link with infection, and this tendency grows stronger as you age. They gave me mega-doses of sulfa drugs back in the day, and now I'm allergic to them. Chemicals in bubble bath powders (remember those?) probably ripped away protective lining in my urethra, and I rode horses in my teens, a contributor to back and pelvic pain problems. In my thirties, a urologist told me my urethra was "too narrow," and did an in-office procedure he referred to as a "ring job," a procedure today's urologists know is totally useless and would like to pretend never happened. Three cycles of the fertility drug Pergonal stirred things up down there as well, so when perimenopause hit—BOOM!

For years, I went through a period of constant antibiotic use—Bactrim, Cipro, Nitrofurantoin, Ceclor—with one UTI after another. I thought my doctors were doing me a favor by prescribing these drugs over the phone without seeing me, and they never made the connection between my diaphragm use and my recurrent infections. Du-uh! (**Because of inappropriate antibiotic use, one in five UTIs is now resistant to some of the frontline drugs used to treat them.**) We used to refer to my diaphragm as "the mouse trampoline," because it was a large, special-order size. Having my tubes tied (no more diaphragm!), Vagifem tabs, and my current estrogen-patch-and-progesterone regimen have calmed things down considerably.

If your urinary symptoms coincide with the hormonal imbalance of peri- or menopause, it's a good bet that you need to "estrogenize" the urethra. See chapters 19 and 21. The localized treatments used for vaginal dryness often work for this as well: 0.5 mg estriol vaginal cream from a formulary pharmacy; the estradiol vaginal ring (Estring); Vagifem estradiol tabs; or Estrace vaginal cream. I was sensitive to the polyethylene glycol, or PEG, in the Estrace cream, and had to get PEG-free cream. Dyes in medications often cause urinary symptoms, so look for a compounding pharmacist for dye-free versions.

Incontinence can often be conquered by Kegels! Remember those exercises you learned in childbirth class, and hold for ten seconds, five sets three times per day. I do them at traffic lights, while I'm brushing and flossing, and whenever I think of them. These are the same muscles you use to stop your urine, so you can tell you're doing it right there, or try to squeeze against two fingers. The supercharged version is a magnetic therapy called Neocontrol (800-895-4298) that contracts the muscles for you. For running and jumping, wearing a tampon helps by keeping pressure on the urethra.

The Absolute Diva of female urology is Dr. Larrian Gillespie, author of You *Don't Have to Live With Cystitis*. She was one of the first to challenge the common belief that various problems with the bladder and urethra were caused by female anatomy – things were "too close together" and "too short" down there, so infections were "inevitable." Dr. Gillespie was one of the first to say "vagina" and "diaphragm" on TV.

Dr. Gillespie stresses that bacteria getting *in* is normal, but problems arise when bacteria can't get back *out*. She urges women with symptoms to get a urine culture done, take a short course of antibiotics *only if bacteria are present*, and come back in a few days and get a repeat culture. **Don't take repeated courses of antibiotics without getting your urine cultured**— this could lead to bladder problems or a chronic condition called interstitial cystitis! (That's what happened to me.) If you or a family member suffers repeatedly from urinary tract infections, you really need to get Dr. Gillespie's book. She warns not to use gobs of lubricant; it's a place for bacteria to grow. Switch from a super to a regular absorbent tampon, and replace it each time you void. If you can "feel" your diaphragm after you put it in, it's probably too large.

Dr. Gillespie's **Pain Control Diet** works well—if you follow it, of course. Coffee, chocolate, orange juice, NutraSweet, carbonated drinks, aged cheeses, and most alcoholic beverages are on the no-no list, along with any other foods high in acid or amino acids like tyrosine. Finnish researchers found yogurt or one cup per day of any unsweetened fruit juice, but especially berry juices, to be preventative. Antioxidant vitamins and Vitamin B6 are helpful, but B12 & B5 could cause spasms or burning.

Cranberry juice can prevent an infection from starting, but is not on Dr. Gillespie's list of helpers for common cystitis. In fact, she warns you to avoid it—and other acid foods like coffee and tomatoes—**when you're having symptoms!** Dr. Gillespie recommends you alkalinize your urine by drinking **1/4 tsp of baking soda in water, take some Tums or other form of calcium carbonate a few hours later, and drink lots of fluids**. This tip works for me, especially if I'm going to a party and having alcohol.

The prescription drug Pyridium or the over-the-counter drugs Re-Azo or Azo-Standard can calm your burning until you get to the doctor. After a fun, sexy anniversary cruise with your husband, you may develop the strong, sudden urges to urinate typical of "overactive bladder" (urgency without pain), a possible manifestation of "honeymoon cystitis." Detrol or Ditropan are useful for these contractions, but an evaluation of the underlying problems is preferable to long-term use of this type of drug. An excellent new treatment for overactive bladder is Botox—a shot stops the spasm of the bladder. Go to a urologist who specializes in women's problems. The young doctor I stumbled onto was mystified by my clean cystoscope, and had no alternatives to the Estrace cream he half-heartedly recommended. I urged him to read Dr. Gillespie's book, but you could see the skepticism on his face; many urologists concentrate on fertility and prostate, and don't know that much about midlife problems.

The Checklist

❏ **1.Water, water, water**—a minimum of 32 oz a day keeps things flowing and glowing! Cranberry or any kind of unsweetened fruit juice or yogurt ward off UTI's when you're not having symptoms.

❏ **2.**Find a urologist who understands the unique problems of women. Put "urogynecologist" in your search engine to find a physician with the dual specialty who understands the interactions of these two systems. You can work backward by asking a local compounding pharmacist (see chapter 21) or try the physician referral at www.ic-network.com. This site is also great to find out about new treatments on the horizon and over-the-counter remedies such as Prelief (against acid), CystaQ (quercetin) for cystitis, and UTI home screening tests for infections.

❏ **3.***You Don't Have to Live With Cystitis*, by Dr Larrian Gillespie; *Screaming To Be Heard*, by Dr Elizabeth Lee Vliet;

For Women Only, by Dr. Jennifer Berman and *The Wisdom of Menopause*, by Dr. Christiane Northrup have great information about urinary and pelvic health. Read these wonderful doctors and **don't consent to any surgeries or procedures until you investigate from their unique perspectives.** (Dr's Vliet and Gillespie have also written excellent books dealing specifically with midlife hormones and weight loss: *Women, Weight, and Hormones*, Vliet; and *The Menopause Diet*, Gillespie.)

23.

Will Power and
Your Financial Diet

*"Have you heard the definition of a woman's needs? From 14 to
40, she needs good looks; from 40 to 60, she needs personality; and
I'm here to tell you that after 60, she needs cash."*
—**Sophie Tucker**

Money is the last taboo for many women, but remember—sex
got a lot better when we started talking about it and sharing
our experiences, and so will our money lives. We can stop
worrying about ending up as a "bag lady" when we take care
of a few important details like credit cards, insurance, savings,
and a will.

Have you heard the one about the frog in the pot? He
won't go anywhere near a pot of boiling water, but if he starts
out in cool water and you turn up the heat gradually, he'll stay
in there and boil to death! That's the way most people are
about credit cards. They wouldn't dream of getting into hot
water by buying a house on their credit card, but they gra-a-a-
a-dually boil themselves to debt with those $30-here-$30-there
purchases. Therefore, **the best safe "investment" in the world**

is to pay off your high-interest credit-card balances. It's kind of like *earning* 20% tax-free and risk-free because you're not *paying* 20%.

Count Credit Card de Balance, the Dracula sucking the life out of your financial security to the tune of over $400 billion, is an ever-present companion from college to the grave. The pizza-and-beer dinner you paid $25 for is $50 after a year on some credit cards; the $1,200 refrigerator you bargained down is $2,000 chilling on the card; and the $4,000 anniversary cruise you took four years ago accrued $3,200 *extra* in interest and compounding costs. A credit card is like a fast-food cheeseburger —they sell the heck out of it, it clogs your arteries (debt), and it's loaded with fat (interest), makes you feel guilty, and does nothing for your health. Resolve that it's *enough*, already, and make this the year you end the insanity!

If you have to carry a balance, shop around for a lower interest credit card on sites like bankrate.com or cardtrak.com. Watch for low rates that will go up because they're only "introductory" and for balance transfer fees. There also may be an advantage to a bank package that includes credit card, ATM, checking, and overdraft and other services. Other credit card tips include:

- **Pay off the credit card bill with the *highest interest rate* first.**
- Make more than the minimum payment often and early in the month to stay ahead of the average daily balance.
- Make credit card, bill, and mortgage payments before leaving on a business or pleasure trip to avoid unnecessary interest, penalties, and black marks on your credit report.
- Debit cards don't offer the "float" (period between purchase and pay) and grace period of credit cards.

Live on your income and not on your "if-come."

If you've made the decision to heal your credit card debt, start your family on a living-without-credit-card program. Have a family meeting and lay it out: designer sneakers, big vacations, pricey sports equipment, coffee bar lattes, restaurant meals, and game and movie tickets are out. Camping, packing lunch, discount stores, part-time jobs, and borrowing videos and DVD's from the library are in. The credit card diet is hard to stick to when your divorced partner is still on a spending spree; the kids may temporarily be wooed away by the cruise and the gifts, but you've got to believe that your love and attention will conquer in the end.

I speak from personal experience on this one. I've said those same stupid things you've said when you're shopping. "This is such a great deal, I can't pass it up!" "We have so much stress right now, and we really need this/deserve this." Scott and I are both suckers for "a good deal." Our mutual area of weakness is our home, where we often find ways to justify fixing up, ripping out, and adding on ("It will improve the value of the house"). Aviva often provides a reality check when I buy something "on sale"; I was exactly like her back in the Age of Aquarius, wondering why my parents needed all that stuff. I'm gradually returning to that mindset, ending shopping as recreation, using actual cash, and forcing myself to delay and think about any non-food purchase over $30. Research shows that 40% of the things we buy are impulse purchases; if you'd invested that money, you'd be experiencing the 25% increase in the NASDAQ this year.

If you're really committed to the idea that credit card debt is a thing of the past, one way to speed the process along is to pay it off with a home equity loan. The benefits are a much lower interest rate that's also tax-deductible, and a consolidation of payments from multiple credit cards into one payment—but there's one huge caution here. This is still your credit card debt and **you must pay off the equity loan and not create new credit card debt**. Zero balance on your credit cards doesn't mean you no longer have credit card debt—it's just moved to a new location.

Now that we've solved the problem, how did we get here? Let's face it—if you haven't been saving, you're probably under the most financial pressure of your life. Automobiles, insurance, tuition, high taxes, a few layoffs, maybe your parents need help—everything is "in your face" over about a fifteen-year period. According to *The Two Income Trap*, the average family today spends *less* of a percentage on clothes and restaurants and *more* on day care, housing, and health insurance. An illness, divorce, or job loss can cause a debt backlog that's hard to climb out of.

I'm adopting a millionaire mentality when I curtail impulse buying, because the wealthy people in *The Millionaire Next Door* drive older cars and describe themselves as "tightwads." They live in homes that average less than $400,000 (in the Northeast and California, a "nice" large house is over $500,000) and have consistently saved 20% of their income. My neighbor across the street, who owns a printing company, is one of these guys. He drove an old Blazer until the day a totally sexy classic Jaguar convertible showed up in his driveway. Sam Walton, zillionaire founder of Wal-Mart, drove an old pickup truck. Millionaires build their security before they buy stuff; that's how they *get* wealthier and *stay* wealthier than the rest of us.

Get peace of mind with Will Power.

September 11, 2001. Thousands of confident, creative, forward-thinking people walked into the lobbies of the World

Trade Center Towers in Manhattan thinking they had all the time in the world to plan their estates and provide for their loved ones. The last thing they would want to happen is for the government to decide who should care for their children and how to split up their assets. And yet, a high percentage of them died that day without a will or trust. How about you, who are so lucky to be alive? Have you done the work required to provide for the people you love? Be ready for the "what-ifs" of life with a will and appropriate insurance, no matter how painful it is to think about.

This is not another thing to beat yourself up about. Two out of three Americans die without a will. Most don't have enough insurance. This is something to put in second place— right after obliterating credit card debt—on your financial action plan. Yes, it's hard to face up to the realities of what happens when you die or get sick, and who you trust to carry out your wishes, but it's another step that helps you own your life.

Assets that aren't owned jointly by you and your spouse could go to a family member you hate, and your Uncle Sam will take a huge and unnecessary tax bite without proper estate planning on your part. Your family could even end up fighting over the care of your children. Financial planner John Sestina warns that a self-prepared will may not be valid or hold up to current estate laws, so hiring a competent attorney (a simple will is about $500), and then reviewing your will every few years, is the best course of action. A high percentage of self-prepared wills are declared invalid. Divorces, second marriages, second families and a family business complicate things further, and a very professional trust is usually needed.

If you want to bet your life's worth on a $30 piece of software, there are some good ones. *Quicken Lawyer 2003 Wills* creates legally binding wills in most states. Questions prompt you as you draft the document, and an on-screen tutorial highlights important issues. Suze Ormond's *Protection Portfolio* contains will and trust forms, credit report requests, checklists of what to do when a loved one dies, an instructional audio CD, access to help on suzeormond.com and other items; you get a few extras if you buy it on QVC. For $55-$115 dollars, *LegalZoom.com* will lead you through a lawyerly set of questions to a will or trust that's legal in your jurisdiction and can be updated at no extra cost. An AARP Legal Services Network Attorney will draw up a simple will for a couple for $100. **A living will/Power of Attorney for Health Care, Durable Power of Attorney, and a letter of last instructions** are other documents to be completed along with your will.

It's your future—insure it!

You have a high risk of suffering a disability that keeps you from working between ages 35 and 65, so check your disability insurance tomorrow. If your employer doesn't pay for it, apply to buy it through them or start shopping for a renewable, non-cancelable, "own occupation" **disability insurance policy.** Use the worksheet on consumerreports.org to determine if you also need a supplemental policy; those who work on commission and many others do. Your 40's and 50's is the time to shop around for an affordable, level (not annual renewable) **15 or 20-year term life insurance policy** to protect your family in their years of greatest need. *Smart Women Finish Rich* author David Bach recommends you have six times your gross annual income, at a minimum. Get in shape for that insurance exam if you want the lowest rates!

If you haven't shopped insurance in the last few years, you might want to check out sites like quotesmith.com, intelliquote.com, and insure.com; professional or social organizations can also offer great deals. Weiss, Standard & Poor's, A.M. Best, and Moody's are the dot.coms to check to see if your insurer is in good shape, while Consumer Federation of America (consumerfed.org) will compare your existing term policy with others for about $100. Many free sites on the Internet like insure.com have calculators to help you figure how much coverage to buy. Organizations like AAA and AARP may give better rates if you buy all your insurance from them—home, life, and car. According to many experts, the optimal age to start paying for **long-term care insurance** is 55, since Medicare covers less than 10 percent of the nursing home costs that 1 in 3 of us will eventually need. The current national average for a year in a nursing home is $40,000. We former recreational shoe shoppers can now use our energy to scout out insurance info on the internet (fair trade? NOT!). If Internet searches are not your thing, ask your computer-geek friend or nephew for help. Reference librarians are also terrific resources.

Get good advice! A financial planner who's a member of NAPFA, the National Association of Personal Financial Advisors, is the best advisor on your insurance, investment, and estate-planning questions since they work on a fee-for-advice basis. Others with CFP or ChFC designations are also professionals, but their income depends on commissions on financial products they recommend; they might favor a "load" investment (with a service charge), because that's how they make money. If you're going it alone, top financial web sites are **Fidelity, Schwab, Merrill Lynch, and E-Trade, Morningstar, and Value Line**—but don't give in to that "time the market and trade often" feeling you get there.

Are you a Baboom—a baby boomer with no savings? Will you be an empty nester with an empty nest egg? People who have no debt, have been automatically saving for years, and have put that money to work in investments in their 20's and 30's can go on to the next chapter. For the rest of us, that "someday" when we would save for college costs and retirement is now (actually, it was yesterday, but now is all we've got.) If you're in that initial empty nest stage, with the kids in college or pursuing new careers, the financial burden can seem overwhelming!

Take the attitude that you're all in this together, being realistic about college choices, living arrangements, and debt. Factoring cost into the college choice teaches a valuable lesson about adult decision-making. "You can go to State U and I'll pay it all, or you can go to Ivy U and pay off a loan for the difference" is a valid presentation of options. You're all adults now, partnering against the challenges of life. All debt is "family debt." All vehicles are "family transportation," interchangeable, unless paid for by one person's efforts. Anyone who reaps a windfall—kid or parent—helps pay down the family debt, i.e. oldest Sis gets the big job and kicks back some tuition cash. The attitude is not "Let Mommy make it all better." The positive midlife attitude is "Let's work on this together because we love and are committed to each other."

Many boomers feel the urge to buy that McMansion they've always wanted, but a dream home is most likely an emotional reward, not an investment. Do you want to be the one to say to your college-bound kid, "Yeah, Princeton would have been nice, but isn't this a great kitchen?" Renting or owning inexpensive housing is so important—about 80% of middle-income homeowners spend more than half of their income on housing in a good school system. Less expensive homes in my excellent school system sell in one day, since smart families know that after the $100 cable bills and $200 cell phone bills are stripped away, you still have to pay the mortgage and taxes. Besides, aren't you just so *over* that huge house?

In his book *Managing to Be Wealthy*, financial planner John Sestina challenges the common wisdom about home ownership when he says "I'm convinced that the **number one reason most people today are behind the eight ball is because they are living beyond their means, usually by owning more house than they should.**" The book's 1986 to 1997 comparison of existing house prices with T-bills and government securities shows those *conservative* investments growing faster than house prices nationwide, blasting the "hedge against inflation" argument for home ownership. In addition, advisers who show naked price **appreciation figures are not showing extra taxes or factoring in the tens of thousands of dollars you've spent improving your home,** one room and one trip to Home Depot at a time. Sestina also recommends developing a home-based business for tax, flexibility, and diversification purposes. It's not how much you *make* that matters, it's how much you *keep*.

Everything You Need to Know About Investing, You Can Learn From Dieting.

Avoid temptation by keeping the junk food out of the house and the check out of your hands.

Money should go into savings first, and then you stretch the rest of your budget to cover. If you plan to "save what's left at the end of the month," you can forget about building that nest egg! Think of it as a monthly bill: you pay your mortgage, your insurance, and Your Future. Start by just saving *something*—stash $2 a day in an envelope in your underwear drawer, just to prove to yourself you can do it. At the end of three months, you've shown you can sock almost $200 away without starving or going naked.

The best strategy is to remove temptation by signing up for your employer's 401(k) or 403(b) retirement-savings plan and have your **contributions come straight out of your paycheck**. You don't agonize over it 'cause you never see it, and your money grows tax-deductible, tax-deferred, and with a possible match from your employer. Outside your employer, start a mutual-fund-automatic-investment plan like T. Rowe Price's for $50 or more per month. Invest your bonus, your raises, your second income, your overtime, your inheritance—any "extra" money that's not in your normal budget should be whisked into your Roth or other vehicle.

Don't get on the scale and measure your waist everyday, and don't check and move your investments often, either.

Chilling out and waiting is how good investing works. Warren Buffett, that boring billionaire from Nebraska, said in an interview to "think of buying stocks as buying businesses, and only invest in stocks of businesses you're familiar with." Of course "Buffettology"—buying companies whose current stock prices don't reflect their true value—requires work and study. Work through your personal finances and read books like *Making the Most of Your Money*, *The Motley Fool Personal Finance Workbook*, *Smart Women Finish Rich*, *Personal Finance for Dummies*, and *The Road to Wealth* to understand the basics of investing.

Buy good companies and index funds with good 5 to 10 year records, though as the saying goes, "past performance is no guarantee of future potential." Ignore most stock-timing advice you see in magazines and on television, and continue to save and invest monthly, no matter what's happening in the stock market. Women are just starting to get this mindset down, developing the steel stomach needed to survive the nauseating swings of today's stock market. An investment club helps too, and commits you to a monthly contribution as part of the group, buying value stocks even in hard times. In the current market, look to get about a 7 percent or above return. Of course, if you have less than 10 years to invest or you're just a jelly-belly when it comes to money, stash it in bank CD's and money markets.

Less than a dozen stock funds have beaten the S&P 500 stock index over the last 20 years, so don't fiddle with forecasters! The stock market is not the lottery, and you won't get rich quick. Other than the occasional Enron debacle or major technology change, it's best to just sit tight through hell, high water, and stock market crashes. If you feel the urge to mess around with your carefully considered investment choices, take a bubble bath instead!

Index funds have out-paced over 75% of actively managed funds because they don't "weigh themselves" too often—they stay in the market, spread the risk, don't do a lot of buying and selling, and, since they're not "managed," they're cheap! Newsletters and brokers who tell you to "time the market" are appealing to your fear or desire for control, but the truth is that **those who invest and do nothing are the big winners**. It's a boring but effective strategy.

Better eat a variety of foods to fire up your metabolism, and invest in a variety of companies to fire up your portfolio. Advisers have warned people for years not to stuff their 401K plans with their company's stock, and the Enron and Lucent situations at the dawn of the 21st century have certainly underscored that notion. Until then, 42 percent of the money Americans put into their retirement plans was in company stock! Take a tip from mutual fund managers—they're only allowed to put 5% of their assets in one company! There's safety in diversity!

Buy large, medium and small-cap funds, international funds– all kinds of stocks and mutual funds that represent the whole American economy, and then the international economy. Before you buy, check the annual report of mutual funds to see if they're too heavy in one area. The tech bust taught us to beware of fads; next time some other sector may go bust.

Don't reward your weight loss with food, and don't spend investment returns. Don't spend the dividends, bonuses, or earned interest—reinvest it right back in those funds! Spending that $100 dividend may seem like a small thing, but planner John Sestina calls this "leakage" a major obstacle to becoming wealthy over the long run! In the last 50 years or so, 87% of the investment returns from the S & P stock index came from reinvested dividends! **80% or more of your retirement nest egg will come from time compounding and reinvestment, not from money you put in.** Let it ride in another IRA, baby!

If the latest diet fad seems too good to be true, it is. If the investment is so hot, it's probably not. Avoid hot stock tips ("I know this guy who works at the company") and a "guaranteed" 20% no-risk return—these will yield the same junk as the pill that burns fat. Why don't people ever learn? The people who get in first often make some decent bucks on the "pump" deal, but the trick is to get out before it's time to "dump" the deal (you won't). Just listen to your mother, the first person who probably told you that if it seems too good to be true, it probably is.

If you don't push yourself, you won't lose weight. If you don't take moderate risks, your investments will fall behind. Parking your long-term savings in money market accounts is like using hourly parking at the airport when you're going away for a month—unnecessary dumping of money! If there's been a 90% increase in showroom prices of cars in the last 15 years, that says you *must* put your money somewhere it will grow *or it will shrink*. In the book *Money Lessons for a Lifetime*, author Jim

Jorgenson writes that: "…using a savings account or money market account to save for college or to build a retirement nest egg is like trying to fill the Grand Canyon with a garden hose. You'll get the ground wet, but not much more. And while you appear to be playing it safe, you're actually running an enormous risk that you'll have less purchasing power in the future than you have today . . .If you are saving long-term for retirement and you don't need the interest income to live on, take the money you have in bonds or bond funds and invest it in the stock market. When you invest in bonds you get about the same sort of price swings as with stocks, yet you miss out on the stock market's inflation-beating returns." Experts used to advise us to start investing in bond funds at 55, but with the new longer lifespan, you may want to look at 60 or so. **You'll live longer and therefore need more money. So you'll have to take some risks and stay in stocks longer,** get it?

Living on earth is expensive, but it does include a free trip around the sun every year. Remember what's free and easy, even as you plan for what's expensive and hard. Loving someone, and them loving you back, is free. The joy of working and seeing the fruit of your work is free. And so many kinds of fun, from feeling the sun to taking a walk to a waterfall, are free. Enjoy!

If you want to reach for the stars, you have to address two factors: money and time. Stop saying you hate financial stuff, and take the baby steps, month after month, to create a financial safety net.

The Checklist

❏ **I. Never Buy a New Car:** some fool's low-mileage lease is your find; 40% of the car's depreciation is in those 1st two years; the $8-to-12,000 average you save can put your savings on the fast track or repay debt; if you buy eight used cars in a lifetime, you've paid off a big chunk of a beach house with that savings!

❏ **2. Get savings out of your child's name** over a year before you sign the financial aid application. Your tax return that the colleges will review for "need" is for the year between January of Junior and December of Senior year. If you could defer "windfall money" to the next year, it might help. Any second dependent in your household taking six college credits or more may **increase your "need" quotient**—check www.ed.gov or www.finaid.org. Look at 529's and Roths to save for college on Morningstar or SavingForCollege.com.

❏ **3.** Not only is college financial aid flattering ("They're dying for me to come there!"), but it's tax-advantaged. For every dollar offered in a grant, you'd have to earn a dollar, plus your tax bracket. Our family loves state colleges, but **private schools have more grant money to give**. Go ahead and apply and see what they offer.

❏ **4.** In your 40's, **consider buying your new 20-year term life insurance policy a year or so before you have to**. You can avoid higher premiums that spring up if those blood pressure and cholesterol numbers spring up! Do not smoke, period! If you quit at least a year ago, apply for nonsmoker rates. Don't lie about your medical history; there's a big database they check with lots of info about you.

❏ **5.** Time to refinance? Does it make sense to convert your IRA to a Roth? Check the calculators on the top sites. The Smart 401K Investing site has the basics and beyond.

Get solid professional advice in addition to net smarts about your 401K when you make a job move—cashing it out, rolling it over, or holding it yourself all have very different tax consequences, so watch out and check with the experts!

❑ **6.** More Americans under 35 believe in UFO's than believe they'll collect Social Security (predicted to go bust in 2017.) The maximum benefit is $1800/month. Can you live on that? To motivate your savings, go to ssa.gov to find out what your Social Security income would be if you retired today.

❑ **7.** Use frequent flyer miles, Marriott points, and other programs and **never pay retail for travel**—top sites are Yahoo Travel, Expedia, and Orbitz. Book air tickets far ahead. Call a hotel after you browse for prices, see if they can do better, and call back again a week before you leave and see if even better rates are available!

❑ **8.** If you need serious credit counseling, use a nonprofit with ".org" in their web address, like the National Foundation for Credit Counseling.

❑ **9.** *Managing to Be Wealthy* is a workhorse of a workbook, a step-by-step, no-nonsense guide to creating a sensible financial plan. With worksheets that help you break down what you want, what you have, and what you need to do to get what you want, it reflects Sestina's 25+ years as the prime mover in fee-only financial planning. There's tons of free, solid advice on Sestina's web site sestina.com.

❑ **I0.** Like the idea of paying bills online, but don't want to pay for the privilege? No problem—Citibank, Bank of America, Bank One, and others have dropped the fee.

The Checkup from the Neck Up

❏ I know what's coming in and I know where it goes.

❏ I pay myself first! I save first, and make the rest stretch to fit.

❏ I have no credit card debt and I protect the future with a proper will and insurance while I invest!

❏ I don't touch my excellent investments. I think of them as a time capsule—I heed good advice, and in 15 or 20 years, they'll be awesome!

24.

Let Your Ripples Loose!
Serving the world, and the kid next door

"Always do right. This will gratify some people and astonish the rest."
—**Mark Twain**

"You must be the change you wish to see in the world."
—**Mahatma Gandhi**

"Never doubt that a small group of thoughtful, committed citizens can change the world. Indeed, it is the only thing that ever has."
—**Margaret Mead**

There's not a long list of things to do at a cabin in Appalachian State Park, but to me and my cousins it was a fascinating place. The woods all around seemed threatening at night when you walked to the outhouse, but during the day the forest was a source of endless piles of sticks for nighttime bonfires and frogs for scaring each other. I loved playing canasta at night with my Mom, Grandma, and Aunt Marie, who was known for throwing her head back in a wild laugh. My aunt wore one of those white bathing caps with flowers on it while teaching me to swim in the lake. My mom taught me too, but sometimes didn't want to get her once-a-week bouffant hairdo crushed and wet.

Other than swimming, my favorite thing to do was to throw a rock or a log into the lake. I loved putting all my dreams into that rock, and throwing it into the cool, dark water. My dreams rippled until they touched all the shores of that big lake. I could imagine touching the whole world with my dream ripple, and that ripple making the world wet and sparkly.

At midlife, we have to come out of the closet with our secret ripple dreams. We've already lived long enough to know that everything we do creates a ripple effect. The Midlife Mama will always have that gnawing feeling that life isn't right until she puts her whole self in to that world-changing endeavor she dreamed of as a child. No matter how successful you are in your professional or family life, your spirit requires that you find somewhere to touch the world with your talent.

Often your vehicle will be something in your past that you enjoyed or were good at, something unique about you, or it may be a whole new thing you've been wanting to learn. Don't feel guilty if it's right in your neighborhood and your girlfriends are doing it, too; it doesn't have to be difficult or inconvenient to be right. It may not be obvious, like "I'm a dentist, so I have to do free dental work for disadvantaged kids." The right thing will pop out like a beach ball held under water. I believe you'll be led to it or you're already doing it, but don't recognize your special role in it yet. When your ripple project starts to click, people will ask you what you're smiling about when you're doing routine things. Planning the next move in your ripple project always makes you smile!

What can we do when the world is such a mess? Against darkness, we can retaliate with light. Osama and Sadaam are still doing their thing, but you and I can build a playground, teach someone to read, or host a meeting to get something rolling. Activist/founder of Share Our Strength and author of *The Cathedral Within*, Bill Shore points out that "Everyone has a strength to share. Often it is a skill or talent they've come to take for granted, but one that can make a difference in the life of somebody else if properly deployed. Mentors share strength. So do tutors, coaches, and doctors…It's not about making your community a better place. It's not about service being good for your soul. It is more fundamental, almost primal. It is what the species instinctively wants to do: to perpetuate itself by leaving something behind; to make a mark that lasts; to make ourselves count."

Start by giving time and energy to people you know. Offer to take the kids while your sister and her husband take a much-needed weekend away. Arrange a schedule of meals with a group of neighbors for the family with a Mom who's getting chemotherapy. Coordinate the family reunion everyone wants but no one's taken the time to plan. Get the lawnmower fixed for your girlfriend who's going through a divorce. Getting yourself out there serving in familiar surroundings is a good first step in fleshing out your ripple project.

Move up to random acts of kindness. Put a letter in the local paper thanking the garden club for their efforts in front of the library. Send a letter to teachers who made a difference in your life or your children's. Get the kids to go through their toys and donate them to a hospital waiting room. Treat absolutely everyone you meet as if they were precious and they have something to teach you. Be as polite and interested in the receptionist as you are in the boss; pass out approval as if it were popcorn, and treat all people great and small as if they were guests in your home. At this point, the direction you'd like to take should be whispering pretty loudly.

Committing to a weekly service "ritual" is like investing – it yields returns far beyond the time you give, because compound benefits build up due purely to your consistency. You feel like you belong there, and you build a trust factor that multiplies your input. A variation on the vital once-a-week volunteer commitment is the volunteer vacation – building a house, helping out in a hospital, or cleaning up a stream with other volunteers during an intense week or two. You travel, live, and work with other team members in the US or abroad, paying a fee to the organizers for putting the whole project together. Habitat for Humanity and its many spin-offs have involved thousands of church groups in helping out here and abroad. The American Hiking Society will have you patrolling the high country, and literacy organizations will put you on a team in Kansas or Costa Rica. This is a real eye-opener for teens and young adults, and they bond with you and other young group members in this energetic atmosphere.

Listen to your anger, that great homing device that tells you the meaning and purpose of your life. Are you angry because the young people in your congregation don't understand your religion, so they're not involved? Heed that alarm called anger, and find out how to turn that around. Thomas Edison wanted to work into the night, so he invented a better light source. Candace Lightner lost a child to a repeat drunk driver and helped to found Mothers Against Drunk Driving—MADD. Worthwhile things happen because someone gets angry. Anger raises the whispers of your soul to a shout and shows you exactly what's calling to you.

The Checklist

❏ **I.** *Get Outside!* is a guide to volunteering for outdoor conservation projects throughout the US. *Alternatives to the Peace Corps lists* opportunities in the US and the Third World, and *Volunteer Vacations* is a general overview of the topic, detailing tried-and-true programs and offering "volunteer journals" to give you a feel for what will happen on your trip.

❏ **2.** Important web sites: Volunteermatch.org, helping you find local organizations that need help; literacyvolunteers.org; voa.org, Volunteers of America programs helping all kinds of people; habitat.org, Habitat for Humanity; and nho.org, National Hospice Organization.

❏ **3.** Got some of the 3.5 trillion unredeemed frequent flyer miles? Donate them to Delta's "Sky-Wish," supporting CARE, United Way, and the Make-A-Wish foundation; and to United's "Miles for Kids in Need" a program that gets sick kids to their medical treatments.

❏ **4.** Maximize your contributions with books like *To Lead is to Serve*, by Shar McBee. This successful non-profit exec shows how to recruit and retain volunteers and gives tips and techniques for successful events.

The Checkup from the Neck Up

❏ There is a specific and divine purpose for my life. I discover more about it every day when I serve God, my family, and the world we live in.

❏ Service makes me larger and stronger, and I lead by serving.

❏ I help others find fun, rewarding ways to give, serve, and get in touch with those who need their help.

25.

News Flash— 90% of Heart Disease is due to Lifestyle Choices!

"Sometimes it's hard for women to relate to heart disease unless they're already suffering from it. It's a silent and initially a painless killer, doing its dirty work in secret and over time. Heart disease can start early in life, even before the age of twenty. In its earliest stages, you can't see it or feel it—it has no symptoms."
—**Nieca Goldberg, M.D.**, <u>Women Are Not Small Men</u>

Cardiovascular disease kills more than half of us—more women than all other causes of women's death combined, including lung, breast, ovarian, and uterine cancer.

In the summer of 2003, two huge studies exploded the myth that half of heart attacks result from bad genes or lousy luck. The studies showed that 90% of heart disease could be prevented or delayed by quitting smoking, reducing cholesterol, and controlling hypertension and diabetes. The ball is now firmly in your court!

After the Women's Health Initiative shot down the heart benefit of the most-prescribed equine estrogen hormone combo, it became obvious that women's heart health has to be addressed in a whole new way. Women generally experience heart attacks 10 years later than men, but a woman's first attack is more likely to be fatal. More women die of strokes than men, and congestive heart failure is more likely to kill or disable women. Women are more likely to be overweight and stressed out, and less likely to exercise. They're also more likely to have a false positive reading from a treadmill test, while a stress echocardiogram screens women more effectively. Triglyceride, CRP, and homocysteine numbers may be more predictive of a woman's heart disease than cholesterol. When we have cardiac symptoms, we're so worried we might "look foolish" or "bother someone," that we're almost twice as likely to die from a heart attack.

There are the symptoms you know:
- pressure or pain in the chest
- sweating, nausea, shortness of breath

and the ones you may not know.
- **pain or numbness in the face, neck, arms, shoulder, or jaw, or back pain**
- **chest or stomach burning like indigestion**
- **unusual tiredness or dizziness**

For stroke,
- paralysis, slurred speech, and dizziness are common, while
- **headaches, disorientation, and pain in the face, arms, or legs** are cues few recognize.

In addition, medical professionals tend to put off ordering

tests and fail to treat women's heart attacks aggressively enough. Unrecognized stroke symptoms mean a woman misses out on brain-saving drugs. If you suspect a stroke, ask the person to smile, raise their arms, and say the words to Mary had a Little Lamb—silly, but it reveals the subtle hot spots.

Girlfriends, God has given us that extra ten years to shape up, since the cardiac cards are stacked against us. We've got to veg out on the greens, whole grains, beans, and fish; pitch the pizza-based diet; and hit the high road with some exercise, meditation, prayer, and positive attitude. We can't enjoy our families and heal the world if we're hooked up to the monitors and threaded with tubes. If we don't care for ourselves, we'll be those little old ladies checking their watches to see if it's time to take a pill.

If you ask some cardiologists, statin drugs will soon be added to our drinking water. (joke) In addition to lowering the cholesterol, triglycerides, and CRP (inflammation) levels in our blood, statins lower the formation of brain cholesterol and the plaques that characterize Alzheimer's disease. Statins seem to lower diabetes and general cancer risk up to 28%, including blocking an enzyme that helps hard-to-treat pancreatic cancer cells spread. The BLI Letter online wrote that:

"The recent meeting of the American Heart Association produced an interesting study…Participants received either simvastatin (Zocor), antioxidants (vitamin C,E, and beta-carotene), or a placebo. The reported results were that antioxidants did not provide any reduction of death due to heart disease or any other cause in this population. The group receiving simvastatin were 16% less likely to die from a cardiovascular event and 12% less likely to die from any cause. Further, they were 27% less likely to have a stroke and 24% less likely to suffer other cardiovascular events."

The study authors made further statements that basically

implied that statins should be used for prevention, not just treatment, of high cholesterol. With some high costs and a long list of warnings from liver and bladder damage to muscle weakness, this approach is not always practical and shows again that health in America is a class issue, with the "have prescription plan" and the "have nots" at odds. But it's understandable why doctors get frustrated and pull out the prescription pad – we just don't do the weight reduction, exercise, and smoking cessation needed to avoid being dependent on pharmaceuticals. Mevacor recently came off patent and can be had for about $30/month. Pravachol is the least likely to interact with other drugs, and Zocor raises HDL while lowering LDL.   And now statins have a new best friend, Zetia, that significantly reduces LDL when combined with the lowest dose of a statin. Americans are getting fatter and drugs are getting better, so I guess you have to thank God they're stepping in when you're not stepping out for your walk.

If you're a "have not" prescription plan, consider no-flush niacin to bring down your L(ousy)DL below 130 when diet, weight loss, ground flax on your cereal, and exercise haven't done the deed. When your LDL and triglycerides are high and your HDL is low, you're a perfect candidate for niacin therapy at about $20/month. Only combine niacin with a statin under a doctor's supervision. Nature Made's Cholestoff uses plant sterols to lower cholesterol for about $8/month, Nutrilite's green tea supplement shows promise, and Solaray's Red Yeast Rice is $10 on Vitamin Shoppe. All cholesterol-busting pills (including statins) should be accompanied by CoQ10. Statin-like supplements may have an effect on your liver, so the liver enzymes and your cholesterol should be tested at your check-up, just as if you were on statins.

The health of your veins and arteries is the key to

successful aging, and the stiffening, thickening, and buildup of plaque in the arteries shuts down the river of life to your whole body. Hypertension, now defined as a reading above 130/85, intensifies the aging process in the kidney, brain, and heart. Everyone knows about heart attack and stroke risks, but did you know that elevated midlife blood pressure predicts memory loss, dementia, and Alzheimer's? Excess salt, sugar, saturated and trans fats, refined carbs, alcohol, and stress drive up blood pressure; fruits, vegetables, fish and other foods with omega-3 fats, aspirin, tea and moderate wine-drinking bring it down. Three hours of walking a week lowers blood pressure, improves artery flexibility, and regulates blood sugar.

A surprise blood pressure reducer is water—the best diuretic of all! The more water you drink, the more fluid your kidneys excrete as urine. The body stops trying to hold on to water, blood vessels relax, and blood pressure goes down. Water bottles stashed everywhere you are facilitate your high water intake. If you feel full and bloated, you're gulping in air with the water, so try drinking through a straw.

Should everyone take an aspirin a day at midlife and beyond? If you have heart risk factors (that's about half of us) or family history, studies indicate that starting at about age fifty, you should start taking an aspirin each day at bedtime, counteracting the early-morning rise in proteins that constricts blood vessels. Lower incidences of leukemia, breast, colon, lung, and esophageal cancers in aspirin-takers are also being studied. A 2003 study showed better results for about half the participants who took uncoated, 325 mg aspirin instead of the coated, low-dose variety. Women with clotting disorders, those taking SSRI's like Prozac, and people taking naproxen and ibuprofen regularly shouldn't use aspirin therapy. Ibuprofen taken within two hours of aspirin blocks its blood-thinning powers.

Don't be confused by recent studies that knocked out **hormone replacement as a heart protector**—these studies looked at only the horse-estrogen regimens like Premarin and Prempro. Evidence that bioidentical estradiol helps the heart continues to pile up, whether it's taken orally or via the skin patch. Dilating blood vessels, increasing "good" cholesterol, reducing plaque, platelet stickiness and blood clots, and facilitating all kinds of free-radical scavenging is the job of estradiol, the most important kind of estrogen. Doctors and patients alike have been scared off by all the scary publicity, but replacing your natural estrogen (see Chapter 20) may be an important step toward your healthy heart.

Results of the 2002 ALLHAT trial surprised many people by indicating that **cheap, old-fashioned thiazide diuretics surpassed newer high blood pressure drugs** like calcium channel blockers and ACE inhibitors. Patients had fewer side effects and better results on the diuretics, though diabetics may do better on Cozaar and those with angina might use a calcium channel blocker.

Over 600 studies have confirmed the benefits of transcendental meditation for lowering blood pressure, and EEG readings of the meditating brain show activity that relaxes the entire nervous system. **Simple belly-breathing while focusing on a word or an object such as a candle work well for blood pressure control for most people who persist and practice over time.** My brain absolutely refused to quiet down, taking off on topics ranging from world peace to what's-for-dinner, so I started using the "instant perfect meditation device," RESPeRATE.

Resembling a CD player on steroids, the battery operated device analyzes your breathing pattern with a sensor strapped around your waist. **RESPeRATE guides you through a 15-minute biofeedback program of breathing** along with the tones you hear on the headphones. When used at least 4 times a week, patients in studies reduced their blood pressure by an average of 14 systolic and 9 diastolic points. That's what it did for me, and you'd have to get a SWAT team to take it away from me now, though the $299 price scared me off at first. The money-back guarantee won me over, and this first nondrug treatment for hypertension to gain FDA approval can be used to complement medication and other therapies. Check it out at resperate.com or 800-509-2389.

> *"Quitting smoking is easy. I've done it a thousand times."*
> **—Mark Twain**

440,000 Americans die each year from tobacco use, and smoking costs $150 billion each year in health care costs and lost productivity. 70 percent of smokers want to quit, 41 percent try, and only 5 percent succeed, according to the Office on Smoking and Health. Don't be discouraged if you've tried to quit and failed; you're in good company. **The average smoker will try to quit at least eight times before they can do it for good. But more than 40 million Americans—three million each year - have successfully quit smoking.**

Increase your chances by addressing the biological, psychological, and social aspects of smoking. Make it a big project, because it is! **Nicotine replacement (the patch, etc) and joining a support group both double your chance of succeeding.** Nicotine patches, gum, and lozenges and prescription nasal sprays or inhalers (which act more quickly) help with the biological addiction using a cleaner, lower-dose form of the drug, but they are not a magic bullet. One-on-one or group counseling or a telephone hotline or internet chat room can help you identify your triggers – stress, meals, socializing, or driving—and avoid them with various strategies ahead of time.

An **antidepressant** can get you through the initial rough spots as well, and increases quitting success for women. You've been dosing yourself with nicotine and you may need to juggle your moods while quitting, so it's all about the brain chemistry, baby. Paxil is reported to have some withdrawal problems of its own, so consider Wellbutrin (same as Bupoprian, fewer sexual side effects), Celexa, or Prozac. **The patch plus inhaler, or either one plus an antidepressant increase success rates.** Plan activities with non-smoking friends, hang out in smoke-free places like theatres and churches, and ask your loved ones to support you. Put an ugly picture of yourself smoking and a list of the many smoking-related health hazards on the frig and taped to the dashboard of your car. Carry around your quit-smoking affirmation and keep a copy of it on the refrigerator, next to the bed, and in your bathroom.

Be very, very nice to yourself for the first few weeks, consciously taking deep breaths and getting plenty of sleep, healthy food, and long walks. **Your body begins to repair itself only 12 hours after you quit.** It's never too late! A woman who quits at 65 gains 4 years, and quitting at 35 nets you an additional 8 or more years of life. I quit 24 years ago while on an organized tour of Greece that included non-smoking plane and bus rides, and my husband and 40 other non-smokers. It was a great way to get through that first ten days of breaking the addiction. **If there's a vacation, sales meeting, or family visit coming up when you'll be away from your usual environment and surrounded by non-smokers, that may be a good 'quit date' to schedule.** Don't you feel like a jerk standing outside all the time, sneaking a smoke?

Midlife Mamas on the Moon

The Checklist

❑ **I.** The American Cancer Society (free phone counsel-800-ACS- 2345), Heart Association, and Lung Association, Nicotine Anonymous, and local hospitals and churches have quit-smoking support groups, and the American Lung Association's program (lungusa.org) is now available online. Call 800-521-2262 or visit medicalacupuncture.org to find an auricular acupuncturist, the kind that works for smokers.

❑ **2.** Angiotensin II receptor blockers, or ARBS, such as Avapro and Cozaar, have been shown to protect the kidneys (important for diabetes patients) and bring down blood pressure without the dry cough seen with ACE inhibitors. Patients given calcium channel blockers (CCBs) had a higher risk of cardiovascular events than those on diuretics and beta blockers. Public Citizens *"Worst Pills, Best Pills"* issued a kidney failure warning on the new statin drug Crestor.

❑ **3.** Chelation has never been shown to halt heart disease or treat anything except heavy-metal poisoning. Don't shell out your hard-earned cash; a study by the NIH on the effect of chelation on heart disease will settle this question. When I hear a pitch for "detoxing," I'm wary – this is a common ploy of modern snake-oil salesmen.

❑ **4.** A Danish study suggests that emergency angioplasties work so much better than anti-clotting drugs for heart attacks, it would be worth a wait of up to two hours for you or your loved one to transfer to a different hospital for angioplasty. Angiomax had significantly better results than heparin in post-heart-attack anticoagulant therapy.

❏ **5.** Overweight, smoking, birth control pills or a recent foot or leg fracture are risk factors for deep vein thrombosis while traveling. Walking the aisles, exercising your legs and feet, compression stockings, or a pre-flight shot of heparin (for high-risk fliers) can help.

The Checkup from the Neck Up

❏ Walking at least 30 minutes a day and eating greens, whole grains, and lean proteins to my heart's content are the foundation of my healthy heart program.

❏ Now that I've kicked smoking, sugar, and bad fats out of my life, I have more energy, I feel alert, and my whole body feels better.

❏ I get my calcium, magnesium, potassium, fish oil, and Vitamin C from high quality sources daily.

❏ When I've made all the right healthy moves to control my blood pressure and cholesterol, I can be consistent with the right medication that's recommended for me.

If the cholesterol number in your blood work is over 200, with an HDL under 35 and/or an LDL over 130, take the Power Foods list to the grocery store and get to work! It is well documented in hundreds of studies that cutting out fat and eating plenty of beans, fish, and fresh fruits and vegetables can lower your cholesterol in a month or less. Concentrate on foods, not supplements.

Power Foods for Controlling Cholesterol

Beans, all kinds including
  soy products
Oat bran
Garlic
Fish—salmon or tuna
Flaxseed
Dark Chocolate (!)
Extra-Virgin Olive & grape seed oil
Avocados
Green Tea

Raw Onion
Almonds, Walnuts, Peanuts
Blueberries, Cranberry juice,
  Bell peppers, Pink Grapefruit,
  Strawberries, Oranges
  (Vitamin C foods),
Apples and Carrots
Benecol and Take Control Spreads
Red wine or dark beer
Oysters, clams, & mussels

Super Supplements for Controlling Cholesterol

Along with a good multivitamin with C, B complex & folic acid, Calcium (1,200 mg with helpers Magnesium, Vitamins D & K, & Boron), and adequate sleep, consider:

Vitamin X- aerobic exercise
  & weight training
Fatty Acids—DHA, ALA, EPA
Coenzyme Q10
Flush-free Niacin
  (inositol hexaniacinate)
Phytosterols as in Cholestatin
  or Cholest-off

Red yeast rice powder,
  as in Cholestin
Garlic
Green tea extract
Chromium
OPC's- pycnogenol
Psyllium Seed
Policosanol (triglycerides)

Watch out for:

Animal, Saturated, Hydrogenated, and Trans Fats found in red meat, butter, margarine, snack and baked goods.

Cholesterol medication interactions with garlic, feverfew, grapefruit juice.

When your check-up shows borderline high-blood pressure (130/85) or higher, try changing your diet and supplements for a few months and go back for a re-check. Consuming less fat and salt and more fruits, fish, and vegetables, can lower blood pressure in as little as two weeks. These foods (not supplements) can also help you lower the level of medication you're taking.

Power Foods for High Blood Pressure

Fish—especially salmon or tuna
Celery
Garlic
Asparagus and All Vegetables
Banana
Nonfat Yogurt

Whole Grains, Fiber
   Cereal- replace refined
Oranges & Grapefruit-
   and all fruits & juices
Extra-Virgin Olive Oil & Flaxseed
Onions

Super Supplements for High Blood Pressure

Along with a good multivitamin with C, B complex & folic acid, Calcium (1200 mg, with helpers Magnesium, Vitamins D & K, and Boron) and adequate sleep, try:

Vitamin X—aerobic exercise
   & weight training
Aspirin at bedtime
Garlic—2, 3x/day
Fish Oil—720mg EPA and
   480mg DHA or more

Hawthorn berry
Coenzyme Q10
Grapeseed extract

26.

What's Up, Doc?
Do your plan your healthcare as carefully as your next vacation?

"A physician claims these are actual comments from his patients made while he was performing colonoscopies: 'Can you hear me NOW?'; 'Take it easy Doc, you're boldly going where no man has gone before.'; 'Hey! Now I know how a Muppet feels!'; 'Doc, let me know if you find my dignity."; 'Could you write a note for my wife, saying that my head is not, in fact, up there?'"

—Internet pass-along

There are times when you have to get ugly with your friends. One of them is when they don't go for their check-ups. As my friend Kathy got closer to her 60th, her "postmenopausal zest" kicked in with a vengeance and she committed to more responsibility at work, taking care of her mother, and planning her kids' weddings, honeymoons, and apartment and job searches. She used to see her gynecologist every year, but since her periods stopped she hasn't seen an MD of any description. Exercise, eating right, and preventive health care were not on her radar screen. I bugged her until she made the appointments for her physical, colonoscopy, and DEXA scan, and after canceling and rescheduling several times, she actually got it all done. Guess what? Her blood pressure and cholesterol numbers are motivating her to exercise, a polyp that could have become cancerous was removed during her colonoscopy, and her bone scan showed she needed to go on medication to prevent further osteoporosis. Kathy showed herself that without self-care, caregivers can become casualties of their own busyness.

It's exciting when a doctor keeps me waiting less that 45 minutes, appears to care about what I'm saying, and remembers some part of my name after my third visit. I had one guy who spoke of my thinning vaginal walls as if they were a remodeling project, and he was amazed when I got tears in my eyes when he pointed out my 20 pound weight gain. The *good* news about doctor visits is that, according to a Rutgers study, they've actually gotten a little longer than they used to be. The study's authors theorize that patients may have more questions to ask because of Internet research. The bad news is that the visits still average only 18 minutes long. The health professionals who authored *Getting the Best From Your Doctor* describe a strategy outlined in the letters **HOPE: H**istorical facts, what you've observed; **O**pinions, how you interpret and feel about the facts; **P**ersonal fears, what worries you; and **E**xpectations, your desires for the outcome of treatment.

In addition to finding a doctor who allocates more time, and **using the expert assistance of physician's assistants and nurse practitioners**, here are things you can do to maximize your visit:

- In the weeks before your visit, **jot down questions** in your planner as you think of them. Check your health insurance to see if you need pre-approval for lab work or if there's a special, direct-to-a-certain-lab procedure.

• Fax or e-mail a **list of concerns** two days before your appointment, with the preface "At my appointment on Thursday, I'd like to talk about…". Make sure you send it to the office your doctor is working at that day.

• Have a list of all vitamins, herbals, and prescription and over- the-counter **medications you're currently on,** in case they're not in the chart. Bring x-rays if appropriate.

• If you're seeing a new doctor, make sure they have your records. Know what to do before a lab test in terms of diet, medication, voiding, whatever (see The Checklist II).

• If the doctor calls you by your first name, feel free to do the same. Don't leave without getting your questions answered.

• If you're getting test results or a diagnosis, bring someone to help you take notes. For serious stuff, absolutely get a second opinion.

Check health facts on medlineplus.gov, healthfinder.gov, healthweb.org, intellihealth.com, Web MD, cdc.gov, ahrq.gov, mayo.edu, drkoop.com, cancer.org, and americanheart.org. If something seems either too good or too bad to be true, check hoaxes on cdc.gov or urbanlegends.about.com.

What is it about men and going to the doctor? It's always "I'll get around to it," or "I'm too busy." I believe the problem lies in the perception that the doctor is in control; your man is not. Let's face it—you get naked and the doctor goes too far south of the equator for comfort. You have to wear a little dress with no back. Can you think of *anything* about that he'd like? And if they "find something," they'll put him in that little dress and wheel him around in a big stroller in a public building!

Have a little empathy, but be firm. Make appointments for both of you on a date he has open, and put it on his calendar. Stress how difficult it is to reschedule. Give a one month, one week, and one day ahead warning (kind of like the ten-minute warning you give your kids.) Remind him about that guy at work who dropped dead and his uncle who might have survived if he'd only…you know. Fear of loss is powerful. You could bring up in a conversation that one of the things you admire about him is that he's not *afraid* to make his health a priority. As a last resort, you could always either promise or withhold sex; it's that important.

You are the lucky lottery ticket for your husband's longevity! Recent studies show that men's number one predictor of good health past the age of 50 is a wife! **In a multi-year study, unmarried men – even those with successful careers – had a much poorer prognosis than married men, though financially independent single women actually enjoyed better health than their married sisters. At midlife, men who have a wife are the guys who have the best life!**

The Checkup Checklist I (with goals)

With your primary care physician annually:
1. Blood pressure—120/80
2. LDL (lousy) cholesterol - < 130 OK, <100 Optimal
3. HDL (healthy) cholesterol - >40 OK, >60 Optimal
4. Total Cholesterol - < 200 mg/dl
5. Triglycerides - <150 mg/dl
6. Homocysteine - < 10 umol/l
7. CRP - <10 mcmol/l

Discuss changes in urine, bowels, energy, sex, sleep, joint pain, alcohol, and recreational drugs. Be honest.

At least every three years, starting at 40:
1. Fasting plasma glucose - >70, <110

2. T(hyroid)SH- >0.4, < 2.0 Optimal, < 4.4 OK

3. Comprehensive metabolic profile plus: ferritin between 60-90 ng/ml to check for anemia or iron overload; and N-telopeptide bone breakdown

Thyroid specialist Dr. Ridha Arem recommends a TRH test for those with symptoms in the "grey area"—2.1 to 4.4.

Between age 45-60—colonoscopy and DEXA bone scan (earlier if you have a family history)

Tetanus/diphtheria every 10 yrs, flu shot annually after 50

Leave check-up with fecal occult test kit after 50.

With your gynecologist annually:

1. Clinical breast exam; leave with mammo prescription

2. ThinPrep pap smear; with PapSure if you have been sexually active in other than a monogamous relationship; with HPV DNA test if you have human papilloma virus (about 60% of us do) or after an ASC-US (abnormal) result.

3. Pelvic exam

4. Discuss contraception, bleeding, fibroids, STD screening, incontinence, sexual habits. Be honest, believe me, they won't be shocked. Also do 1-7 of above blood screening if you don't see a primary MD.

African-American women must grab their sisters and get these tests; 30% greater risk of death by cancer is caused by a lack of screenings. Ask about the new test for ovarian cancer if you have family history—Atairgin Technology's LPA blood test, more accurate than CA125. Contact them to be in the clinical trial and go on wcn.org to assess your risk.

Be sure to get that thyroid test if you're suffering from weight gain, dry skin, constipation, and other common midlife complaints—new result guidelines have been set, and you may need a touch of Synthroid to get your metabolism to where it should be.

> Sometime between age 40 and 53, get serum levels of all your ovarian hormones on day 1 to day 3 of your cycle, day 5 to 7 of the placebo week of your birth control pills, or anytime if you've had a hysterectomy or no longer menstruate. Do it first thing in the morning before a pill or right before a new patch if you're on hormones. At minimum, go for:
> 1. estradiol - above 90/100 pg/ml
> 2. testosterone - 400-600 pg/ml (40-60 g/dl)
> 3. progesterone - luteal - 5-25 ng/dl, follicular - 0.1-0.4 ng/dl
> 4. FSH—above 20 mIU/ml means low estradiol/menopause
> Test guidelines and optimal ranges from It's Your *Ovaries, Stupid!* Elizabeth Lee Vliet M.D, but she stresses that the "optimal" ranges are where *you* feel well.

See a dermatologist to have your spots and speckles checked. I showed a suspicious one to my primary and he said it looked OK; a dermatologist later biopsied it, found a squamous cell carcinoma, and prescribed Aldara cream. My point is, regular docs can't always spot (ha!) this stuff, so get a skin check, with mole mapping if need be. Don't be surprised; they need to check places the sun don't shine (genitals) and the most common trouble spot for women is the legs. Find free screenings in May and June on aad.org, cancer.org, or skincancer.org.

Right after your big physical, you may be going to the drug store to fill your new prescription, or you may be helping your parents with their prescriptions. CAUTION: If you don't have a prescription plan, there are many options to save money. (Even if you do, you can save deductibles by filing three months at a time.) You can check out US mail order prices, try a generic version of the drug, or use an older, less expensive brand in the same "class" of drugs, like Lipitor (take CoQ10 with it) instead of Zocor, or Prozac instead of Celexa. Recent studies showed, for example, that inexpensive thiazide diuretics were more effective in lowering blood pressure than expensive newer medications. See if your drug has a generic at theunadvertisedbrand.com. My local supermarket pharmacy charges $138.00 for thirty 20mg Zocor tabs. A Canadian pharmacy, myPrescription.com, had it for $2.05 less per tablet.

Is it safe to order from other countries? With a million Americans buying drugs from licensed pharmacies in Canada, not one complaint about fake drugs has surfaced. Regulated as closely as US pharmacies, they display a license number, require a doctor's prescription and your medical history, and provide an address and phone number in addition to their web address. A quality-standards accreditation agency, IMPAC, has begun a list of pharmacies you can depend on, beginning with CanadaDrugs.com. Drug maker GlaxoSmithKline has stopped supplying its products to Canadian pharmacies that sell to Americans, and the battle will continue until some compromise is found.

Then you have to **keep a close eye on how you're reacting to any medication or supplement you're taking**. I wish I could print my friend Jo-Anne's whole story, but here are the highlights. After a blood pressure check at the local pharmacy sent her to her doctor, she started taking a blood pressure medication daily, with her vitamins. Two years later, she noticed she was crying frequently, and at public events she would fill up tissues when no one else was crying. When her doctor dismissed it as just "being sensitive," Jo-Anne carried on until three years later, when she found herself depressed and unable to function, right after moving to a new state. She tried ten different antidepressants, each one feeling like "an elephant sitting on my chest," until one finally worked, and she took it daily with her blood pressure pill. Another year went by, and Jo-Anne was concerned about all the medicines, so she saw an allergist who told her she was allergic to the blood pressure medication! All the years of tears, six years of down moods, and finally the depression—so easily dismissed as a "midlife crisis"— were because of a medication! Though the symptoms came on slowly when she started the drug, the depression and anxiety cleared immediately when she went off it, and she's found a natural supplement that keeps her blood pressure under control.

When doctor and lab bills roll in, check the charges. **Always appeal a denied claim**, as it may turn out it was just coded wrong, mistaken as optional, or they sent it to the wrong insurance company. Our recent bills all bounced back, as the entire family was put on my daughter's COBRA instead of just my daughter. Often someone in the doctor or dentist's office is "the claims meister," who can go to bat for you. Company, local, and for-pay healthcare advocacy groups can help you uncover errors and get coverage.

The Checkup Checklist II

❏ **I.** Schedule a mammogram, clinical breast exam, or self-exam about a week after your period ends, when your breasts are least tender. Have the clinical exam before your mammo, so your ob-gyn can alert the technician to pay attention to any questionable areas. Don't use deodorant, powder, or lotion. An MRI picks up 94 percent of invasive cancers in dense or high-risk breasts, versus 78 percent with mammograms. Look for another new test, CAPP, in 2004.

❏ **2.** Go for a pap smear in the middle of your cycle to avoid blood in the sample. Refrain from sex for 48 hours

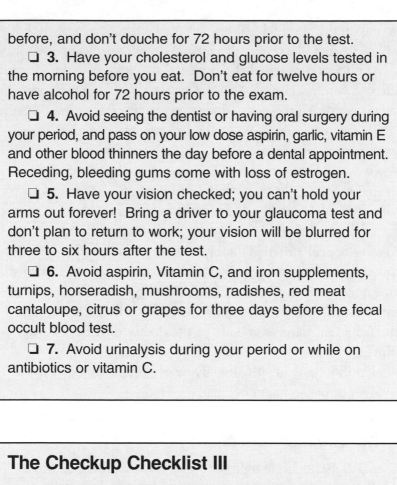

before, and don't douche for 72 hours prior to the test.

❑ **3.** Have your cholesterol and glucose levels tested in the morning before you eat. Don't eat for twelve hours or have alcohol for 72 hours prior to the exam.

❑ **4.** Avoid seeing the dentist or having oral surgery during your period, and pass on your low dose aspirin, garlic, vitamin E and other blood thinners the day before a dental appointment. Receding, bleeding gums come with loss of estrogen.

❑ **5.** Have your vision checked; you can't hold your arms out forever! Bring a driver to your glaucoma test and don't plan to return to work; your vision will be blurred for three to six hours after the test.

❑ **6.** Avoid aspirin, Vitamin C, and iron supplements, turnips, horseradish, mushrooms, radishes, red meat cantaloupe, citrus or grapes for three days before the fecal occult blood test.

❑ **7.** Avoid urinalysis during your period or while on antibiotics or vitamin C.

The Checkup Checklist III

❑ **I.** Smokers or former smokers should get the spiral CT scan instead of an x-ray—it detects much smaller tumors and boosts survival.

❑ **2.** The Triage Cardiac System or Triage BNP will diagnose heart attacks or congestive heart failure in 90 minutes, versus the former long confirmation.

❑ **3.** Much faster diagnosis for oral cancer—Oral CDx.

❑ **4.** The IBD-CHEK identifies Irritable Bowel versus Inflammatory Bowel with a stool sample instead of colonoscopy or barium enema. A new Mayo Clinic stool test that spots pre-cancerous polyps will soon make colonoscopies a tool for removal, not diagnosis.

❑ **5.** Know Lyme disease for sure in 20 minutes with the PreVue blood test.

❑ **6.** New tests on this list are from *Health* magazine—stay up on the latest!

You deserve the finest healthcare—take the time to get it!

27.

Boning Up For Your Future
Osteoporosis—Be afraid, be very afraid

"I've been taking calcium and exercising for 20 years—I can't
believe the test shows osteopenia!"

"My doctor wouldn't authorize the DEXA because I'm only 42,
but the back specialist insisted. Guess what?
Osteoporosis is the cause of my back pain."

"I didn't realize my thyroid medication put me at risk."
"I broke a wrist at 48, tripping over a garden hose.
The test showed bone loss."

"I'm afraid to walk the dog, carry heavy groceries, move garden
plants around, or walk in the dark—and I'm only 54."

"What a jerk I am! My mother's bones are in better shape than
mine, because she took care of herself.
I'm even afraid to join my church softball league."
—Comments from an Internet chat room

Sticks and stones can break your bones, but ignorance will
hurt you the most. I hope you know about calcium, but did
you know that your body only absorbs about 35% of it? You
probably know about exercise and weight training bone

benefits too, but have you "gotten around to it" yet?

• Starting around age 35 we lose up to 1 percent of our bone mass per year, and in the first years after your period stops you may lose up to 5 percent per year!

• 77 percent of women who have osteoporosis don't know they have it, so they aren't doing anything about it.

• Almost 20% of American women 18-25 have low bone density, 50% of women over 65 have osteoporosis, and 89% of women over 75 have it.

Complications of osteoporatic hip fractures kill more women every year than breast cancer, and you have a one-in-three chance of suffering from osteoporosis in your lifetime. The sad thing is, we know from other cultures with different diets and habits that *simple steps could bring all these percentages to zero*.

At 30, the battle of the bone begins.

The best time to prevent osteoporosis is when it's the farthest thing from your mind, but that was in your 20's so you only have now. Your bones are a beehive of activity through your entire life, with the Pac-man bone-eating osteoclasts digesting the old bone, while the osteoblasts build new bone. As you age the 'blasts build less, and when estrogen declines at menopause the Pac-man drilling overtakes the filling, your bones start to look like swiss cheese, and bone mass declines. The only way to know who's winning—the 'blasts or the 'clasts—is to get a DEXA scan.

The bone-builders need calcium to do their thing, and we lose 200 to 300 mg of it each day in urine, stool, and perspiration. In addition, our intestines absorb less calcium as we age so we need to take in 1,200 to 1,500 mg a day. What type of calcium? In recent studies, the conclusion was basically that **calcium is calcium—don't get fancy**, just take about 250 mg three times a day, in addition to your multi with calcium and vitamin K, and get the rest from food. If your supplement dissolves in vinegar, it will dissolve in your stomach.

Because it's easier to digest, I've started taking my calcium citrate/magnesium/D horsepill early in the day to avoid, shall we say, the "gaseous emissions" sometimes caused by the calcium carbonate/magnesium/zinc/copper/manganese I take after dinner. Wheat bran and other high fiber foods cut absorption of calcium, so keep the intake spaced apart a bit. **Calcium-fortified orange juice is a calcium bonanza—it's already dissolved, the natural sugars and acid in OJ help boost absorption, and you get vitamin C and potassium.** Viactiv Calcium Chews with D and K are a nice little 20-calorie chocolate treat. Then there are some very advanced calcium sources in liquid and pudding form—they're called milk and yogurt and they work great in your body because the co-factors like vitamin D and lactose have been put in there by the designer who created the universe. Milk with added protein and calcium packs an even bigger punch. A low-fat moderate-protein diet, potassium/magnesium foods like bananas and blueberries, soy foods, and tea are bone smart, and the supplement ipriflavone inhibits breakdown and aids bone building, especially paired with calcium.

Hip, Spine, Hooray!

Exercise doesn't just maintain hip bone, it *increases* it. Squats and leg presses really help the hip, and the more weight you lift, the more the hip benefits. Actor Christopher Reeve had the bones of a 100-year-old man four years after his accident, but an electrically stimulated exercise regimen brought his bone density back to normal. If he can do *that*, what can *you* do?

Replacing estradiol (see Chapter 21) using skin patches like Climara and Vivelle DOT does a better job of building your spine, and **the combination of all three—calcium, exercise, and estradiol—does the best bone-building job of all.** Prempro and the other equine estrogens that were shot down by recent studies didn't do the best job of bone retention for many women, in addition to their breast cancer and heart disease associations. Progesterone skin creams haven't shown the bone benefits of estradiol, but oral micronized progesterone has shown results. Very low-dose testosterone for women also helps, and men with low testosterone do get osteoporosis.

Fosamax and Actonel used post-menopause with estradiol boost bone preservation more than either therapy alone, and are excellent on their own in their once-a-week dosage. I am one of those smaller-framed women who probably built less bone to begin with, but I was absolutely shocked when my 50th birthday DEXA scan showed me at only two clicks above osteopenia! That darn Evil Inherited Tendencies Fairy struck again, so now I've got the Actonel/Vivelle thing goin' with my calcium and exercise routine. I have no extra bone to lose! NSAIDs like Celebrex and Vioxx slow bone healing, while thiazide diuretics used for high blood pressure help conserve calcium in the kidneys. Breast cancer drugs Evista and Tamoxifen have been shown to inhibit bone breakdown.

The Checklist

❏ **I.** To see if your bone meds are working, use the NTx test of second morning void urine. The number should be lower than 35. You can also use a bad number on this inexpensive test to justify a DEXA scan to your insurance company.

❏ **2.** The bone formation drug Forteo could do a lot of good for those with fractures or a lot of bone loss, but warnings have been issued that the drug caused tumor growth in rats during trials.

❏ **3.** Estradiol replacement will help bone loss in the jaw and periodontal disease; you'll notice less gum bleeding and tenderness.

❏ **4.** No, the phosphorus in soda doesn't interfere with calcium absorption—there's ten times the phosphorus in skim milk as in soda. Just don't let teens drink soda instead of milk.

The Checkup from the Neck Up

❏ I enjoy low-fat dairy products and green leafy vegetables and leave my supplements out where I'm reminded to take them.

❏ A brisk walk outdoors in the sunshine four or five times each week strengthens my bones and provides vitamin D.

❏ An effective weight training program provides so many benefits to my body, and I feel my flexibility and balance improving with my healthy program.

28.

Your Laugh Lines Prove You've Had More Fun Than Your Kids!
Is Mom Visiting You Everyday— in Your Mirror?

"This is where I am now—smack in the middle of my forties. If I had to sum up the decade so far, I'd say this is definitely the "oh shit" decade…Your forties is when you finally start coming to terms with things you can't change—and figure out how to improve the things you can…"In your fifties, more than ever, if you take care of yourself, it shows (and if you don't, it really shows)."
—**Bobbi Brown**, from <u>Bobbi Brown's Beauty Evolution</u>

You're in a paradox in your 40's—part of you thinks you're still young, while your image in the mirror may say you look okay until you put in your contacts. You try to strike a bargain by eating the perfect diet, exercising, and entering the mad world of Maintenance, with a capital M. Or you surrender and become best friends with the pizza delivery guy, Krispy Kreme Donuts, and a "nice, neat short haircut." You realize it's true that men "age better" than women, because their skin is thicker and they exfoliate every day when they shave. In your 50's, you've got to break out of your fashion rut—pigtails, Farrah's frosted shag, and the faded jeans your husband likes are not a "signature look." If you wore a trend the first time, you probably shouldn't wear it in its latest incarnation. Be aware of that fine line between chic and Alice in Wonderland that can be avoided by having a hair stylist who tells you the truth. As you get closer to your 60's, you may meet your girlfriends for lunch and notice you're all wearing turtlenecks, scarves, or stand-up collars to hide "the neck problem." No one wants to reach for the bread basket for fear of revealing "the hand problem."

The sexiest, most attractive move we can make is to forget contorting yourself into something you're not, do the up-to-date self-care, and be fully engaged in life! I love saying what's on my mind instead of being an edited version of myself. Yes, when I see myself in photos it doesn't match my mind's image, and sometimes I'm loud and large and "too much," but the person saying I'm too much usually wants everyone over the age of 40 to disappear. We can't be paralyzed by the expectations of others or the myths we haven't overthrown. No generation of woman has lived the second half we are about to live; the look has been hinted at, but not set by Sophia Loren, Sigourney Weaver, Barbara Walters, Diane Sawyer, Tina Turner, and Angela Bassett. The successful second lives *we* lead will change everyone's perception of what a person who "looks that old" can do.

Don't compare yourself with magazine photos—top models like Cindy Crawford and Clotilde admit they hardly recognize themselves in those photos because they've been so digitally altered and retouched. If you have some version of Adobe Photoshop on your computer, even you can make skin brighter, eyes larger, and waists thinner. When you see Goldie Hawn and Susan

Sarandon on the big screen, remember that the makeup and hair people just stepped out of the shot. Their "people" turn them out for red carpet events. Cher—well, she must have the best genes and the most extensive maintenance program in history, but hey, the image lives. Rock stars now have digital tuners that bring their voices to the right note during concerts and recordings. My point is that media images are not real, and it's just ridiculous to hold yourself to a standard that doesn't even exist in real life!

"I have the skin of an 18-year-old; she'll be so mad when she sees how wrinkled I got it!"

A star makeup artist behind the model's runway, Bobbi Brown reveals that she's a midlife mama just like you and me in her book *Bobbi Brown's Beauty Evolution*. She celebrates all women, from beautiful young models to hang-gliding 87-year-olds, and has some basic recommendations for 40- and 50-somethings:
- a really good haircut and the stuff to style it
- a slightly heavier moisturizer
- a yellow-toned, translucent, light-reflecting foundation that disguises redness
- under-eye concealer that's one shade lighter than your skin right up to your lash line and into the corners of the eyes
- black mascara and shadow lining the top and bottom lids
- a little brighter blush and lip color with liner.
- Less is usually more and blend, blend, blend.

Shaping the brows and finally learning to use the eyelash curler before the mascara are other midlife eye-opening strategies. To learn how to do the Pamela Anderson "smoky cat eye" and other looks, go to makeup411.com. A spray-on tan from Mystic or Hollywood Tan looks awesome in the summertime, and the fine mist of that technology is your foundation of the future. Similar to the airbrush wand used in nail salons, our personal compact airbrush systems will put a long-lasting, wrinkle-defying layer of micronized foundation on the skin. It's available at Barneys New York for about $500, but I'm visualizing a small appliance for about $40 in your future. Meanwhile, a can of aerosol spray foundation or bronzer already exists—Era Face or Era Rayz on classifiedcosmetics.com or by calling 866-372-3223.

At about $20 a spritz, the spray-on tanner booth can get a little pricey. To use regular self-tanners effectively, choose the shade based on your skin tone, not on the color you desire; light/medium ladies need light/medium tanner. Exfoliate all over with a scrub in the shower, use a light moisturizer if you need to, and apply the tanner when you have some time to dry, while folding a big pile of laundry and matching some socks on the bed perhaps. Dab the knees, heels, ankles, and elbows to get some of the tanner off. After your base coat, you can reapply every three or four days, using your fake tan to cover the vein map of New Jersey highways on your legs. Discount brands, Clarins, and Estee Lauder sprays work well, and a salon product called Fake Bake mousse does a better-than-average job. Lemon juice, whitening toothpaste, and hydrogen peroxide lighten self-tanning mistakes and chlorine gives your fake tan a mottled look.

Natural ingredients beat high-tech fou-fou.

Back in the 80's, skin care ads showed scientists mixing up skin care products in the lab—what my girlfriend Audrey calls "high-tech fou-fou." Now the rage is ingredients from nature or enhanced substances from our own bodies, with **antioxidant vitamin C** one of the evident winners. A polyphenol cream made from green tea is being tested to fight skin cancer. Copper, kinetin, soy, biotin, CoQ10, grape seed, green tea—all kinds of nature-derived creams are out there touting their skin-firming benefits. C-Cellex, Lancome Vitabolic, The Body Shop's Vitamin C Protective, and Neutrogena Healthy Skin all have topical vitamin C, but the only verifiably stable version is Artistry Time Defiance Vitamin C & Wild Yam. You break the seal on the C, mix it, and use it up within 30 days—very potent and motivating!

Sloughing off the dead skin cells using **retinol** (synthetic vitamin A) creams while stimulating the skin's own collagen to grow is the next best thing to the tretinoin Retin-A, Renova, and hydroxy acid peels prescribed by doctors. Estee Lauder's Diminish, Artistry Alpha Hydroxy Serum Plus, and ROC creams use fruit acids to peel, while Artistry's Skin Refinishing lotion uses an oat-protein complex that's safe for the most sensitive skin. The latest prescription "slougher" is **tazarotene cream or Avage**, which seems better tolerated than Retin-A by many kinds of skin. **Non-ablative lasers** are the newest skin-smoothers in the dermatology office, doing a "controlled burn" that smoothes the skin without the visible sunburn and skin-shedding of other laser treatments. All these products and procedures make the skin more reactive to sunlight, so vigilant sunscreen use is called for.

What you *put in* your body surely counts as much as what you *put on* it, with the fruits, greens, whole grains, and lean proteins winning out again. Eating lots of fiber and omega 3 fats glows up your face just as surely as potions and creams. Dr. Nicholas Perricone, author of *The Wrinkle Cure*, has created an effective shortcut with his weight- and inflammation-reducing diet of salmon, egg whites, and vegetables and fruits. His treatment products use DMAE (derived from salmon), vitamin C ester, alpha lipoic acid (ALA), and tocotrienol vitamin E. Daily and evening versions of Renewal Crème at nutrivera.com also include these ingredients, plus small amounts of progesterone and estriol, the weak estrogen.

Bioidentical hormone replacement addresses the loss of collagen under the skin and hair loss due to hormone imbalance. The patch and progesterone regimens described in Chapter 21 will have a favorable effect on skin and hair, and may also solve the dry eyes that trouble midlife contact lens wearers. Better skin, sleep, sex, mood, memory, and vascular health – these benefits of a typical bioidentical patch-and-progesterone regimen must be balanced against the fear of all hormones fostered by research on the horse estrogen regimens. Dr. Northrup mentions good results from a formulary pharmacist's blend of 150 mg of estradiol and 1,500 mg of natural progesterone in a 10 oz bottle of fragrance-free Jergens lotion. One teaspoon a day spread on the face improves the skin while providing hormone replacement. The online Hopewell Pharmacy commonly fills prescriptions for 3% estriol face cream, while HormoneProfile.com makes available .5 estriol/progesterone face creams without prescription.

See Spot run when you use Tri-Luma, a prescription cream combining tretinoin and hydroquinone that's used for melasma and other large dark areas on the skin, while Solage is designed for smaller sun and age spots. Non-prescription versions include Artistry's Bright Idea and Shiseido's Whitess. Vitamin K creams help those prone to bruising and Mederma from the drugstore can speed the healing of scars and stretch marks.

Zits—at my age?

Adult acne reflects the fact that midlife is kind of like being a teeny-bopper—you can't figure out whaaat the heck is going on with your skin! Calming the complexion storm with birth-control regimens like Ortho Tri-Cyclen, Ogen and Diane 35,

and Yasmin gets to the probable root of acne after 40—
hormone changes.

The ClearLight high-intensity light kills the bacteria that
cause acne, and the ThermaCool TC radio frequency
treatment improves both acne and wrinkles. Prescription drugs
Differin and Tazorac work for many, and the Proactiv line is a
gentler, non-prescription solution with a money-back guarantee.
Who'd have thought there'd be a need for mass-market
products like Neutrogena Anti-Wrinkle/Anti-Blemish and
Aveeno Clear Complexion Moisturizer, but they're available
pretty much everywhere. Witch hazel and alcohol are out and
salicylic acid is in for midlife toners, and tea tree oil is a gentle
antibacterial ingredient. For the pimple that inevitably grows
right between your eyes or on the end of your nose before an
important occasion, apply an ice cube for three minutes, a clay
masque product for five, and then wash off. Do not squeeze!

The bumps, pimples, and redness of **rosacea** are a whole
other story, and a new prescription gel called Finacea has been
added to the topical and oral antibiotics and use of lasers or
pulsed light sources already used by dermatologists. The
intense pulsed light (IPL) zaps squiggly blood vessels, tones
down redness, and reduces flushing. Topical vitamin C and
betaine HCL taken orally are other useful therapies for rosacea.

Let's talk teeth, those pearly predictors of other health
problems like heart disease, osteoporosis, and diabetes. First,
the toothbrush—make it a rotation oscillation electric
toothbrush like the Braun Oral B Plaque Remover. Add a
bacteria-fighting mouthwash and get it together with the
flossing routine. Use Atridox antibiotic patches before your
dental cleaning to reduce bleeding and gum pockets. Pay for
an extra cleaning-only visit each year in addition to your
check-up, especially if you take antidepressants – the dry

mouth can cause extra decay. Get on a payment plan with a good dentist to take care of too many dark fillings, gaps, or a high gum line. Home whitening is okay, but getting the custom-made bleaching trays made is a better investment, since your teeth will need to be lightened about every two years. Use Sensodyne toothpaste for a few weeks to get ready for lightening, and ask for Gluma desensitizer if you're really sensitive. BriteSmile and Zoom whitening take the smile 4 to 7 shades lighter in one sitting, but they're expensive and will also have to be repeated every two years. A great smile overcomes a lot of obstacles!

> *"Let's face it—if I see something sagging, dragging, or*
> *bagging, I'm going to pluck it, tuck it, or suck it."*
> —**Dolly Parton** on *Larry King Live*

Well, let's add "fill it" to your list there, Dolly, because the latest way to deal with wrinkles is to fill them with Botox, Restylane, Radiance, Cosmoderm, Artecoll and other forms of high-tech spackle that will pretty much replace collagen over the next few years. Let's say you want to be looking good for your daughter's wedding—you get rid of the fine lines with non-ablative laser therapy; fill in those vertical lines on top of your lips with Radiance or Cosmoplast; plump up your cheek bones with Perlane; blow off the deep crease between your brows and crows feet with Botox; and suck out that extra chin with a little, tiny bit of liposuction. (Well, now you've heard my wish list.) The ThermaCool technique heats the lower layers of the skin without a visible burn, causing the collagen fibers to shorten and achieving results similar to a surgical lift. None of it involves months of recovery time or the "wide mouth bass look" sported by a certain older comedienne, but it does involve thousands and thousands of dollars. Maybe all this will be old hat for our daughters at midlife, included in their annual physical or whatever, but for most of us it's only a dream. (Okay, I admit it—I filled out an application for the Extreme Makeover television show.)

Have you been curious about skin resurfacing and plastic surgery, but afraid to visit a doctor? No problem! One of America's most respected plastic surgeons, Dr. Gerald Imber, has made his popular book The *Youth Corridor* available FOR FREE online at drimber.com. It's the 2003 edition, it's updated continually, and he answers readers' questions. Imber, master of many procedures but known especially as the youthful neckmeister, agrees with most doctors that skin creams available without a prescription are all mildly effective for maintenance; just use one that feels good, regardless of "special" ingredients. He gives a thumbs up to Renova and other AHA creams, and urges caution regarding human growth hormone. He notes that laser resurfacing gives slightly better results than chemical peels, but is more expensive.

For a more comprehensive look at the less invasive options, read *The Non-Surgical Facelift Book* by doctors Byun, Mendelsohn, and Truswell. Though these procedures are often called "lunch time" facelifts, many involve at least a week of "don't-leave-the-house" recovery. *The Smart Woman's Guide to Plastic Surgery* has especially good info on liposuction and breast implants. If you want the humorous slant, check out *Two Girlfriends Get Real About Plastic Surgery* from two who've been there and know a lot about that. It's important to do your research before you go for a consultation because:

- you get better answers if you're more specific and knowledgeable
- doctors tend to recommend what they've been trained on or the $10,000 laser they just invested in and

- all kinds of M.D.'s are doing this stuff because it's cash, not insurance, so you want to be sure to use a top pro.

Speaking of top pros, The Insider Man Tells All in Dr. Bob Kotler's *Secrets of a Beverly Hills Cosmetic Surgeon*. He gives the straight scoop on the superspecialization of plastic surgery, and reveals the importance of computer imaging and the details of safe operating rooms. He even talks about negotiating fees with your surgeon and watching out for hidden fees!

Will we soon be walking around with frozen faces that show no emotion? Are we disrespecting our struggles and joys by erasing the lines that express them? If we wipe the anger off our faces, will it be stored somewhere else in the body? If our faces reflect our souls, will our souls be less rich if we erase the face?

Questions to ponder…but we can know one thing for sure. If a woman wants to remodel her body or her face, let's not whisper or judge. Just because you've had your eyes done doesn't mean you're not spiritual. Fixing something that's bothered you all your life may open up your whole attitude, ability to serve, and ability to love and be loved. Maybe you've worked through some challenges and you just want your outside to match your new inside. Whatever it is, it's your decision.

The Checklist

❏ **I.** The new "midface lift" is a "pulling up" from the mouth to the brows, instead of the old "pulling out" to the ears lift. The result is smaller incisions, a cleaner jawline and a refreshed look that doesn't look tight. Have you ever stood at the mirror and pulled everything on your face up? That's basically what Dr. Gordon H. Sasaki does, using Gore Tex fibers to tighten the area just above the jaw, attaching to a below-the-skin anchor above each ear. This no-bandages, no-recovery procedure costs about $4,000 and takes the Loma Linda University surgeon about an hour.

❏ **2.** Raptiva may be the miracle injection you've been waiting for if you have psoriasis. Diflucan, known for yeast infections, is a safer "off label" med for nail fungus; warnings about liver and heart complications have come out about Sporanox and Lamisil, the "official" drugs for nail fungus. Cold Sores Begone and Canker Sores Begone are herbal answers to these pesky sores.

❏ **3.** In a ten year study, graduate students looked at photos of 45-55 year olds and judged who looked youngest. The ones they picked turned out to have had 50% more sexual intercourse than those who looked their age. Make love, not wrinkles!

❏ **4.** If you want to know the latest and greatest about health and appearance innovations, get *Health* magazine. Just when you've been wondering about something, they've got a list of the ten best ways to do it.

❏ **5.** Grind your teeth but can't afford the expensive night guard? Get the adjustable SleepRight at splintek.com for about $70. UltraWhite %16 teeth whitening (about $120) on Yahoo.com sends you the mold material and the custom mold is made in a lab, just like the dentist's.

The Checkup from the Neck Up

❏ I realize that my appearance affects how people see me, but I know that my actions and attitude are more important.

❏ Knowing there's a 50% chance that a melanoma the size of a dime has already spread, I am diligent with sunscreen and check for changes in my spots and speckles.

❏ My self-care is balanced and appropriate—I have friends who are good role models and my internal compass tells me when I need to ramp up or scale down.

❏ A focus on living a happy life that matters comes easily to me and I share that attitude with others.

29.

Loss—Getting Beyond "Why Me?"

"If I wake up and feel down and sad and depressed, I cancel everything for the next day or so. I don't take a shower, and I don't wash my hair. I don't even leave my bed except when nature requires me to. I grab two bags of potato chips, I pull the covers over my head, and I lie there feeling sorry for myself. I weep. I curse. I suffer—not just a little. A lot. I suffer as much as is humanly possible. I suffer more in two days than most people do in a year. I do everything I can to make myself feel as bad and sad as possible. Nobody throws a pity party like I do."

—**Linda Richman**, remembering the loss of her son in her book <u>I'd Rather Laugh</u>

On a lazy summer day, wearing shorts or a swimsuit, you may have played the game of "This is how I got this scar." It's easy to talk about it now because the frightening accident or surgery that caused it in the first place is over. You've lived to tell about it, and you can share the details in a pleasant conversation, letting the summer sunshine warm that once-scary spot.

You can form a tough, strong attitude around your loss like the tissue around a scar. A key element is—how will

you explain your loss, to yourself and others? How will you talk to yourself about it? Could you speak with joyful tears at the funeral of your 23-year-old daughter, like my friend Debbie? After her daughter's two-year losing battle with cancer, Debbie explained Kelly's life and death in a triumphant way. Yes, Kelly's life was way too short, she said, but look at all the wonderful experiences and friendships she crammed into it! Look at the fantastic people attending this funeral from all over the world who knew and loved her, and the patients and healthcare professionals she inspired with her optimism and strength! As the family slogs through the year of "firsts"—first Christmas, birthday, Mother's Day—they continue to interpret Kelly's life as one that was well lived, instead of constantly lamenting what she missed and how much they miss her. Living in fear, anger, depression and regret can lead to a "poor me" existence, and recovering alcoholics, for example, say that "poor me" leads to "pour me another drink." Striking a balance between honoring the past and allowing yourself to hope for a great future is the main task of grief.

What does strength after loss look like? I think it looks like arms reaching out for help and understanding, a person who is able to say "I can't do this by myself." It looks like my friend Pam, who was consoling others after the sudden death of her beloved husband Danny. As each shell-shocked friend walked into her living room, not knowing what to say to her, she embraced us and allowed the tears to come. Feeling better but a little foolish at the role reversal, we were now ready to smooth *her* feathers when they would ruffle up in fear. Her wholeness, spirituality, and tremendous family allow her to take one step at a time in her new life without Danny. A long-established exercise habit and some *I Love Lucy* videos help relieve stress, and she surrounds herself with people who are quick to point out everything that is positive about her past, present, and future. Yeah, she gets mad, sad, and upset. But without making a big deal about it, she is one of the most spiritual people I know. *"Don't you get it?"* her glowing smile seems to say, without the need to lecture anyone about her spiritual independence.

What's her secret? Why does everyone want to get next to her, instead of avoiding her and steering clear of the confrontation with her tragic loss? It's simple. **She has everything she needs inside her, and nobody can take it away. Her peace and happiness come from the inside, and she doesn't need anything that she doesn't have.** She really believes that Danny is in a better place and that God's plan is right, even though we may not understand it. Intelligent, sharp, and resilient, she's aware that other people fear her situation, and she even jokes about it. When a group of us were playing carnival games, with the husbands winning stuffed animals for their wives, Pam joked, "Won't somebody win one for the poor widow?" Her self-awareness is amazing, especially since her husband died such a short time ago!

Living with a long-term disability and the loss of a healthy body can be even tougher than a death—the maintenance and hard work lasts a very long time and can wear down even the hardiest of souls. Relationships tend to go one-way or the other, with some families torn apart by bitterness and anger and others shining with the grace of commitment. My friends John and Jennie Belle illustrate the attitude of commitment, with a loving decision to live an awesome life despite John's paralyzing injuries from a burglary/shooting. Their self-discipline, successful habits, and legendary love for each other are an inspiration to all who know them.

In the past, men showed strength by covering up their pain, while women would share with others and fully explore pain. Now men are also being empowered to connect with others and shed the cowboy image. Police, firemen, and rescue workers wept openly in the aftermath of September 11. It's now routine for athletes to embrace each other, eyes glistening with tears, after a victory or a defeat. A man may cry out to his mother while driving away from her grave, and all who hear feel privileged that they were trusted enough to share in that raw emotion. Instead of "fighting against" the terrorists inside and outside of our bodies, on good days humanity seems to be moving toward an acknowledgement that we can be strongest when we recognize and share loss, and live a connected life, knowing that life is short.

If you are grieving or comforting those who grieve, you set the tone. **You choose whether to say "He suffered for so many years" or "He really enjoyed playing cards with his friends, didn't he?" As always, the words you speak will tell your brain what direction you want to go in.**

Grief comes in one size—Extra Large

"Letting it out," speaking some of the dark thoughts you've had during a long illness or immediately after an accident, has to happen at some point. Talk to a trained counselor, such as a therapist or member of the clergy, or tell the person you're venting to how you want them to react. People with no experience of grief just don't know what to say or do to help you. Forgive them. **"I don't expect you to solve my problems or teach me not to hurt, but it would be a big help if you would just listen,"** you could say. This is actually a handy phrase to pull out of your brain on many occasions, so keep it where you can find it.

The Checklist

❏ **I.** When someone you know suffers a tragic loss—just be there! No excuses! Don't add the pain of being avoided to a horrible event. "I can't handle it" or "It makes me uncomfortable" doesn't cut it. Stop whining. Sign the register, send a sympathy card, but hold your long letter until later. Offer to do practical things like pick people up at the airport or provide food.

❏ **2. Things NOT to say at the death of a child:** "You can always have another baby." "Well, at least you have_____ (other children) to keep you busy." These phrases imply that the child they lost was replaceable. Just say, "I'm sorry." Pay special attention to brothers and sisters; Mom and Dad may not be as available as they might wish. Children need to know what has happened and fully grieve, just like adults.

❏ **3. Things NOT to say at any funeral:** Don't ask detailed questions about the accident or illness, imply that the care they received was not optimal, or comment on the appearance of the deceased. Not everyone believes that this death is part of God's plan, "it was his time," or that the person "is in a better place." If the family wants to talk about these things, just listen. Follow their lead in talking about the lost loved one, and don't be afraid to mention happy memories. Sometimes if you break the ice, they can feel more comfortable talking about the good times. When photos are displayed, that means that's what the family wants to focus on.

❏ **4.** Allow them to express their grief and don't pass judgement on "dredging up all that stuff," or when they should be "over it," "go out more," "take it easy," or exercise. Continue to offer support through all the holidays and "firsts", respecting their need to socialize *and* their need to be alone. Stay in touch with the bereaved via e-mail if you kept in touch that way in the past.

❑ **5.** If you are the person grieving, try to live as balanced a life of work, play, and contemplation as you possibly can. Many describe plodding numbly through life, taking it one day at a time, trusting that at some point life will hurt a little less. A glimpse of joy won't mean you've forgotten your loved one; it will mean that joy is a normal part of life. Find a support group at, webhealing.com, Widownet.com or Youngwidow.com, and use *The Widow's Financial Survival Guide* in settling the estate.

❑ **6.** Share this checklist with teens and young adults when appropriate; they have never confronted these situations before and need to know how to act and what to think.

The Checkup from the Neck Up

❑ I am a helper and comforter to all who are dealing with loss, including myself. My faith is a powerful healer.

❑ Life can be tremendous after loss if we choose to see it that way.

❑ I place no rules on anyone, only love, on healing from loss.

30.

Start From the End and Look Back
When you have to decide what's really important, it's usually what you already have.

"I'd get up in the morning, do my exercises, have a lovely breakfast of sweet rolls and tea, go for a swim, then have my friends come over for a nice lunch. Then I'd like to go for a walk, in a garden with some trees...In the evening, we'd all go together to a restaurant with some great pasta, maybe some duck—I love duck—and then we'd dance the rest of the night. I'd dance with all the wonderful dance partners out there, until I was exhausted. And then I'd go home and have a deep, wonderful sleep. That's it."
—Morrie tells what he'd do with one healthy day in <u>Tuesdays with Morrie</u>, **Mitch Albom**

People who are very ill are experts on what's important about life. Knowing that your time may be limited makes you look back and catalogue the joys you've already experienced and prioritize the time you have left. It's interesting that most people with a serious diagnosis don't take off for Hawaii or that world tour they've been putting off. Instead, they tend to stay in their normal surroundings, sharing simple, precious time with loved ones. When you have to decide what's really important, you usually discover it's what you already have.

Terminally ill patients don't worry about dying; they only wonder if they've lived enough.

Women who've been ill teach us that we *can* be replaced, thank God! They've had their knuckles smacked with a big stick by the circumstances of illness, and somehow *others* get the laundry, job, shopping, and kid and pet feeding done. They've slowed down and let themselves heal. You can hand the overstressed life or illness over to God, and the other tasks to *anyone* who'll take them. We *can* give ourselves time to focus on health and happiness and the world still turns. The phone rings and no one answers it, the grey hair shows and no one colors it, the e-mail comes in and no one reads it—the world turns without your input, and if you're lucky, you can offer some hugs, smiles, and phone calls in return. After your mental vacation or your healing, you can just pick up where you left off. Be there for others when you can, and the seeds will come back as fruit.

Vibrant people on the high end of the lifespan also focus on the beauty of living everyday life. It's kind of annoying— successful, happy people in their 80's and 90's all say the same thing. "Look on the bright side, stay involved in life, work at something you love, exercise and eat moderately, enjoy life, family, and friends," they all say. I think we call that "wisdom."

It's hard to focus on the simple pleasures when your 9-year-old is failing in school, your deadline at work is looming, your husband isn't talking much after being passed over for a promotion, your semester-abroad college student has mono in Spain, and your period lasts for 21 days! If Advil and Tums have become new food groups for you, where do meditation and prayer fit in? How can you enjoy life when your to-do list is three pages long and you're in debt? What steps can you take to be a happier person and overcome the messages you learned as a child—"You're not good enough, you don't deserve it, you're not lucky, pretty, or smart?"

Simplify and delete—what to cut?

When there's fifty zillion gigabytes on your computer, it just won't take any more! You can't put anything else in there until you delete, delete, delete! Life is the same. **If the system is about to crash, you must simplify your life.**

After 9/11 and during the war in Iraq, many of us got into the habit of watching CNN or checking the cover page on our search engines 24/7. But we have to realize that news organizations thrive on what's wrong and threatening. They discovered years ago that their ratings went up when they reported on horrifying personal tragedies (mother kills child) instead of important world issues (nuclear arms talks). Is it any wonder that many people find they feel less anxious and sleep better when they **cut down on obsessive news watching**? At the very least, you'll have more time to stoke up your supply of emotional energy with positive reading, going for a walk, catching up with a friend, or working in your garden.

How do we get out of the mindset that it's good to constantly work, think about "the next thing," and cut corners to save time? An effective strategy might be to **discover the value of one day** without anything to do except rest, relax, and enjoy loved ones. Think about it—one day with no TV-watching, meal preparation, car travel, errand-running, chores, computing—nothing but talking, napping, reading, strolling, sharing simple meals, and really listening to each other.

An intentionally simple day that is different from other days is a tried and true concept in many religions, but a high art in Sabbath-observing Jewish households. Shabbat has been called "an island in time," a day when a community walls away distractions of all kinds to concentrate on worship, family, and rest. It is credited with a low divorce rate and successful family life among observant families. The concept can easily be adapted to your family; **you could request Mother's Day, your birthday, or a visit with close family to be a simple, no-media day of walks, naps, hanging out in the yard, sitting down to eat together, and lingering over the table to catch up on what's happening in all of your lives**. Don't ask me why, but this seems to be easiest to accomplish when you go camping, stay in a cabin, or when you're at a pool, lake, or the beach. For some reason, everyone seems more willing to relax in these settings, so by all means designate all or part of your vacation as a no-activity zone. Keep the wireless devices away and gently pull back the family member who's drawn to the TV.

There's a whole "simplicity movement" afoot, and it even has it's own lovely magazine—*Real Simple*. It's all about the universal realization that **time is precious and "stuff" gets in the way**. It's a change that characterizes both those who get laid off or went down with the dot.coms, and those who are suddenly successful, buy a bunch of "stuff,' and realize that stuff doesn't make you happy. The book *Your Money or Your Life* was the first of many excellent books that ask if stuffing your ever-larger house with stuff is making you happy, and outlines a program to drain some of the materialism from your life stream. Put "simplify life" into the Amazon search engine, and you'll find a ton of books that help you answer questions like **"What is 'enough' for me?"** You quickly realize that a *simple* life is not *easy* and it's not about depriving yourself of stuff; it's about making space for what's really important.

The truth is so obvious at midlife—stuff expands to fit the space available, it becomes invisible after you have it for a while, and too much stuff can even hide the stuff that's really important. **Getting out of the Acquisition Mode and into the Appreciation Mode** is an important over-40 task that is a natural part of the midlife transition. I still love to look at extravagant homes and over-the-top cars and jewelry, but I recognize they don't fit in with the priorities I've worked so hard to discover.

God has a bigger dream for you than you could ever have for yourself—but how about giving God some specifics to work with? We all know that writing a list of our dreams and goals has power. Finally knowing what you want brings you closer to it and to God. Why do we put it off? Do we think we're unworthy or greedy? Do we secretly believe that if we touch our dreams, they'll break into little pieces? Perhaps we don't want to write it down because we're afraid we'd have to act on it and we're frightened. Writing down your goals sets forces in motion that will help you reach them, forces outside of you that can help you. Just *knowing* your goal starts a process of selection at every turn in life's road—will this help me reach my goal or not?

A very effective way to flesh out your dreams and goals is to keep a journal, a process that you may have abandoned when you put aside your pink Barbie diary with the little gold key. Today, it's a major self-discovery tool used in colleges and professional workshops, and journaling is certainly cheaper, and possibly better, than seeing a shrink to sort things out. Forget the "shoulds" and guilt trips when you're writing in your journal; write in it what, when, and how *you* want to, though morning writing is the best for many. Perhaps you could start with a list of blessings that you add to each night, kind of a never-ending thank-you note to God for all your good stuff. It feels personal when you write in the present tense (Today I), about *feelings*, not events, and include details and random serendipities. Inevitably, some negative thoughts will intrude, and you can put these in a separate section to park your worries and explore them. (Writing them down also wrings the fear out of them.)

You can keep a spiritual journal, where you record insights from what you're reading, prayers, or personal conversations with God; let it be your personal "wailing wall." Use your journal to transform or renew professional goals or solve workflow and time concerns; writing things down makes possibilities pop out.

My friend Tom used journaling to stop the cycle of anger he learned from his father. "I didn't realize until I was forty that I had inherited my father's inability to handle personal hurts, disappointments, and anger. Though I appeared happy and positive, my temper seemed closer to the surface and affected my relationships. At a real low point in my life, I ran into a man who exposed me to journaling. As I started to write letters to God, my thoughts exploded onto the pages. The more I wrote, the more things became clear to me. My anger subsided, my marriage became fun again—it was like a mental enema."

Tom shared his journaling experience with his son Brian when he noticed that Brian exhibited the same anger-stuffing behaviors in shouting matches with his sister. The next night, Brian told Tom he'd written for over an hour about his feelings toward his sister and others who'd really hurt him. Tensions around the house lessened dramatically, and in a matter of weeks the kids were laughing and talking about things. "Since that time, my son and I have grown much closer. We talk about everything and we've stopped the cycle of anger in our family."

The Checklist

❏ **I.** The aim of Michelle Weldon's *Journaling to Save Your Life* is for you to realize that your life is worth preserving on paper and that journaling is do-able. An abuse survivor, she's "been there" with the bad and the good and helps you with exercises that get you unstuck from the overwhelming blank page.

❏ **2.** Don't be so focused on self-improvement that you forget to have a real life. Having some events to look forward to on your calendar is more important than washboard abs. If your inner child is writhing around in pain, maybe she just needs to have more fun!

❏ **3.** The world's most extensive spiritual journals are the books *Conversations with God, I, II,* and *III.* Learn from them how to talk to God, how to trust your experience as a form of communication, and discover that God wants to know who's listening!

The Checkup from the Neck Up

❏ I live my life on purpose, with purpose; I don't waste time worrying about what I "should" do.

❏ I honor and celebrate my past, live enthusiastically in the present, and actively choose my future.

❏ Faith helps me see that my life is huge and I'm not defined by my past or present circumstances.

❏ They tell you to put your oxygen mask on first before you help others; getting to know my priorities first helps me serve others better.

31.

Have a Thick Skin and a Thin Heart—Forgiveness Lets You Live More Fully

"Experience has taught me that when we treat ourselves like cherished souls, a divine source supports our efforts…When you take steps to honor your Self, like starting a journal, asking for a well-deserved raise, or saying no to unwanted demands on your time, you'll set in motion a higher order in your life. And the best part of all is that you don't have to believe in the magic of grace to reap the rewards. Just take good care of yourself and wait for the miracles; they'll become a very special source of motivation throughout this journey."

—Cheryl Richardson, Life Makeovers

Jamie always seems angry about something. Her blue eyes blaze at any perceived invasion of her belief system. She attributes all her problems to the mother who abandoned her, and details her mother's horrifying, unforgivable actions to any one who'll listen. She's proven herself to be the absolute Top Dog Victim at her support group. Her pain and anger are a big part of who she is. But here's the sad part—her mother's been dead for ten years.

Who gets hurt by all this anger and pain? It's obvious that the only victim is Jamie. Now think of the terrible thing that was done or said to *you* by someone with the power to really hurt you. I'll bet it didn't take you long to think of it. Your heart beats faster, your eyes narrow and the whole injustice of it all comes crashing down on you again. Your feelings for that person give you permission to have a pity party for yourself and feel superior or self-righteous. But that grudge also steals your health, your peace of mind and your ability to move forward. As Dr. Phil would say, "How's that working for you?"

I had one year of college under my belt when my parents asked me to come home because they couldn't afford college any more. The family business had gone bankrupt, my father had a stroke, and college tuition had to get in line after food and a roof over our heads. I worked a day job and a night job, contributing to the household and stashing any extra money in the safe at home. I wanted desperately to go back to school and my boyfriend (Scott). One day when I looked in the safe, I discovered my parents had "borrowed" my money without asking me. When Scott flew down to visit me, my parents started a shouting match that made it clear that they had also been opening my letters from Scott and reading them.

It took me years and years to even begin to forgive them. When you've seen your parents as powerful and righteous, they've got a long way to fall off that high pedestal. My parents hit the hardest of brick walls, and their fall was not graceful. They were probably embarrassed to ask me to borrow the money and planned to return it, and they were investigating my relationship "for my own good." Later, when I applied for food stamps to supplement my college scholarship, I discovered they were claiming me as a dependent for tax purposes, even though they were not supporting me at all.

I didn't take a big "risk" to reconcile with them, insisting on bringing out the details of everything they had done wrong. We never really confronted the issues. I just decided at some point to forgive and forget. I think they realized from my actions and my words that I just wanted to love them. **By forgiving them, I was not condoning their actions.** They were responsible for their actions, and they had to answer for them to God. **I was taking back my power from them by letting go of my anger. After that, I created boundaries that made it unlikely they could really hurt me again. They had to live with their choices;** true peace of mind may have been hard for them. They may have rationalized what they did, but that doesn't concern me. Once in a while, all these years later, I still get angry, but I remember other times when they supported me and I appreciate the sweet, happy life they gave me to grow up in. In later years, I often reminded my parents of all the wonderful things they did for the family when they could—helping my grandparents financially, hosting elderly relatives at the holidays, taking us on vacations, and supporting us in school activities.

People who've been physically and mentally violated far beyond my experience have forgiven. You don't need that person's cooperation to forgive and they don't have to say they're sorry. Learn from Dave Pelzer, whose tale of appalling abuse by his mother is detailed in *A Child Called It*. Like him, you may have to forgive the same person over and over again. But do it, because feeding and caring for that grudge will poison that sweet juicy strawberry of the rest of your life.

In *Letters to a Young Therapist*, Mary Pipher, Ph.D. writes that she was trained to ask "What have other people done to you and how do you feel about it?" The result of this question is endless discussion about Mom's criticisms, Dad's indifference, and their unfair focus on your talented brother. Pipher, a sweet-spirited leader of the positive psychology movement, *now* asks "What have you done for others, and how does that make you feel?" She contends that focusing on what *you* can do *now* gives you more control over your future than rehashing the past.

Acknowledging where you've come from can help you understand the knee-jerk reactions you exhibit that later result in me-jerk recognition. Why do I always freak out when he compares me to my mother? Why do I forget to call him when I know it makes him crazy? Some self-examination can result in an apology and a promise to change that includes a well-thought-out plan to improve your response.

But once the family drama has been explored, the stuttering behaviors scoped, and the motivation understood, can we move on to the fun part—actually living? Instead of constantly asking why, move directly to "what." Not "Why would he do that?" but "What is my next move?," "What can I do to avoid that next time?", and "What choices does this open up for me?" An examined life is important, but a life of repetitively re-examining the same patch of grass is irrelevant. Time to get a life, forgive, accept, and move on!

Instant Forgiveness—Kicking it up to the stars!

I have a new concept that I'm really getting a kick out of— instant forgiveness! We have instant microwaved food, instant Internet access, instant satellite positioning—why not instant forgiveness? Your father embarrassed you by getting belligerent with a waiter? The whole family agreed in advance to laugh about it, he does it all the time, and you've forgiven him in advance. You can always count on your sister to compare your kid unfavorably with hers? Instead of clenching your teeth and not believing "she's doing that *again*," you all get a huge kick out of it because you've shared the observations and you forgave her before it came out of her mouth. You embarrassed your daughter by repeating a confidential story? You apologize, pick up your foot, and wiggle your toes in your mouth, because you've already forgiven yourself!

Instant forgiveness has given me so much freedom, because everything is "like water off a duck's back" – it rolls right off and you never dwell on it. I'm sure people who value worry and picking out the negative aspects of everything think I'm just stupid, but I'm so *happily* stupid! Things that used to bother me are now like wind beneath my wings, as I fly with power and vision above the junk that used to fill my mind and focus on the sweet unseen spirit beneath the irritations of life. What a rush, when you blink and the stink is gone! Try it!

The Checkup from the Neck Up

❏ When I forgive *you*, I am releasing *me*!

❏ I take the high ground in all my interactions, believing the best about people's intentions.

❏ I respect and appreciate the lessons I've learned from disappointment, and I choose to accept rather than judge.

❏ Instead of wondering why people do things, I wonder what my next move is.

❏ I have taken back my power by letting go of my anger.

32.

Keeping the Faith
BIBLE = Basic Instructions Before Leaving Earth

When I was a kid, I noticed that people got more religious
and read the Bible more, as they got older.
Now I realize they're studying for the final exam!

At the halfway point in her life, it only makes sense for a
Midlife Mama to examine where she's been and where she's
going. One of the central questions of midlife, "Is that all there
is?" must be dealt with, so we can feel free to throw ourselves
into the second half! As a child, sitting in a holy space, you
may have resonated with the rituals, the candlelight, the music
and the shadows of sacred things. Then you grew up, got rational,
and became one of God's frozen people, setting aside the experience
of faith for more "intellectual" pursuits. Living in a spiritual no
woman's land, you may feel lost when midlife bares its teeth
and you've lost that childlike connection with the miraculous.

Whether it's a personal brush with illness or divorce, caring
for aging parents, or the 9/11 World Trade Center disaster,
midlife events often provide a wake-up call for those who've

wandered away from their spiritual lives. There's a need to believe that a higher power is in control of life, that we can trust God's timing instead of seeking instant answers. We hunger for God's gentle cues, guiding us like a skillful dance partner so that our lives really flow with the music. Most of all, we need to believe that we are basically good and that God cares for us. If we can actually trust that a more powerful force values us, then we have something we can depend on.

Boomers will boost the ultimate self-improvement program.

78 million boomers, always a generation of seekers, will become increasingly spiritual as they age, like their mothers before them. People describing themselves in polls as "religious" increase from about 30% at 18 to 50% at 65, with women more likely than men to do so. It's natural, girlfriends; don't fight it, celebrate it! Researchers have even taken snapshots of the over-40 brain in a mystical prayer state. The part of the brain that draws the line between the body and the world shows a dramatic reduction in activity. Apparently we're hard-wired to experience spiritual feelings and the reality of our connection with the rest of the universe.

Finding your spiritual self can parallel another familiar process, according to Marianne Williamson, author of *A Woman's Worth* and *Everyday Grace: Having Hope, Finding Forgiveness*, and *Making Miracles*:

"Spiritual growth is like childbirth. You dilate, then you contract. You dilate, then you contract again. As painful as it feels, it's the necessary rhythm for reaching the ultimate goal of total openness. The pain of childbirth is more bearable as we realize where it's leading. Giving birth to our selves, our new selves, our real selves, whether we are men or women, is a lot like giving birth to a child. It's an idea that is conceived, then incubates. Childbirth is difficult, but holding the child makes the pain worthwhile. And so it is when we finally have a glimpse of our own completion as human beings…when we do, our hearts finally melt. Our rage transmutes. Our burdens are released. And that is our birth into who we really are. It's messy and painful and noisy and big. But it's all that matters, and it's all we're here for, to chuck these stupid clothes we wear, of false ambition and pride and fear, and come out naked and beautiful and new."

I believe that *every* path that leads to God is valid. Whether your prayers come from the Bible, the Torah, the Vedas, the Tipitaka or the Book of Mormon, they will lead you to becoming a better person. Most of my prayers consist of thanking God for my many blessings and asking for guidance in understanding why things happen. *Traveling Mercies* author Anne Lamott claims the best two prayers she knows are "Help me, help me, help me" and "Thank you, thank you, thank you," top categories in everyone's prayer inventory. Even if you start with a pick-up line by saying, "I don't know you God, but I'd like to," and continue from there, any words you're comfortable with will travel from your mouth to God's ear. *Anything* is better than giving God the silent treatment!

Be open to spiritual moments in everyday life. In writing this book, I would often feel compelled or inspired to write about something—as if I was being led to serve you with that subject. I would pick up a book, looking for something, and a really important idea would be there. Simple, huh? It comforts me in a way I can't describe, but there it is. I feel a little weepy as I write this, because faith has always been so easy and natural for me, and I know that so many people struggle with it. Thank you, thank you, thank you.

Stressing your muscles and cardiovascular system causes you to grow in strength and endurance. Spiritual discipline in everyday life works the same way, with right choices and consistent study increasing our capacity to hear God speak. **Listening to God—instead of looking inside yourself—may be the shortcut to the meaning of life.** Think about it: if God created you and revealed the process in the bible, you already have your Owner's Manual. Adding service *really* empowers the spirit, generating an inner force we can use to attract mentors and flex our faith muscles. Plus, it makes you feel great and expands your vision of what *you* can really do to help God perfect this world.

All major faiths command you to live a healthy life in order to serve God!

In the old and new testaments, there are over 100 passages commanding you to do this. The person who skips exercise and eating right because they're so heavenly-minded can soon become no earthly good! You can't serve God, the world, your family, or yourself if you don't do what it takes to support the body that supports your spiritual energy. The world's greatest renewable energy is there for the taking, and it's yours if you'll only look for it. And spiritual energy—that un-self conscious goodness that makes you feel connected and lets others feel they've been heard and understood—supports every uplifting change you and your family want to make.

You may be skeptical about matters of faith, but the pursuit of a spiritual life is worth struggling for, even if all you look at is the numbers. **Those who attend religious services have a seven-year higher life expectancy**, according to a nationwide study of 21,000 people from 1987 to 1995. A Duke University study of 4,000 adults found that **attendance at a house of worship is related to lower rates of depression and anxiety. Better recovery from surgery, lower blood pressure and fewer health problems overall have been documented in other studies.** Unfortunately, studies also show that the fastest-growing group of those answering religious-affiliation surveys are those who answer "none."

In the new millennium, there is a growing group of people who identify themselves as belonging to a religious group, but they don't belong to a congregation or affiliate with any organization. Translate that to mean, "In my heart and mind, I identify myself as a Christian/Catholic/Jew/other, but I just ain't *goin'* there." There're about 30% more adults who *identify* themselves as belonging to a religion than those who are actually *members* of an organized group. Regardless of whether this is due to the crazy busyness of our lives, the variety of faiths within families, or an intentional attitude about organized religion, it is a fact. I've been in this group myself, sublimely free of organizational fundraisers, the need to teach Sunday school, and the religious school car pool.

I received a forceful message that there was something missing at the funeral of my friend's mother. She had been a member of her congregation in the Bronx, New York for 30 years, watching many ethnic groups and pastors come and go. Yet, the young pastor currently shepherding this flock wept openly when she expressed the sadness of the entire congregation that this bright spirit would no longer be sitting there. "Who will lead *my* memorial service?" I asked myself, "Will it be someone who barely knows me, who gathers appropriate material to write an emotionless essay?" I had to admit that in my current unaffiliated state, the answer would be yes.

Join the world's longest-running book club!

Investing—time, money, and emotional involvement—in your spiritual community is like investing in any other team you belong to. There are financial drains and annoying people who drag the team down. But how can you really refine your jump shot or your drive to the basket without playing with others? After you work through scales and other musical basics, how can you learn to improvise jazz if you're playing by yourself? The same principles hold with your spiritual life; how often have you dozed through a familiar service, only to be startled by that one flash of insight offered by the most unlikely person? As the congregation slogs through the yearly round of bible or Torah readings, will you be forced to read a passage that has a surprising insight for your life? You don't get to choose which book to read, but discussing the meaning of that one *important* book can be a benchmark for the rest of your life. Would you throw your head back and sing with all your heart if you were praying at home? And yet it's precisely that simple act that may transcend all the metaphysical discussions you've ever had.

Start with the religious tradition you grew up in. Don't run off and become a Buddhist because you think you can snatch some quickie peak experiences. Look at the faith of your mothers from an adult perspective before you throw it in the trash; you may be able to recycle it into a journey you never imagined. You may still have "issues" with many of the teachings you learned growing up, but I often hear people say they're able to interpret them differently through the filter of their life's experience. Try hanging your intellect on a hat rack for a few months and experiencing the familiar rituals, melodies, and holidays with your emotions and a child's wonder. Stop judging and relating your faith to your old family circumstances, and just "be" for a while. See how that feels.

If you went where your parents pointed you when you were growing up, it may not feel right to you to **"shop around" for a spiritual home.** Today it is common to do this, however, because your success in fitting this into your life will depend on how strongly you want to "connect" with this congregation. Like exercise, religious observance is great if you'll only *do it,* not just join a certain congregation because the car pool is convenient. Today's savvy kids will notice if they're the only ones in the family showing up. Interestingly, though, I've seen kids from nonreligious households join a congregation as part of their "rebellion." Religious school schedules, location and costs, and the vitality of the teenage youth group is a big concern when children are involved, but take some time to actually go to a service before you sign up. Does it feel uplifting and comfortable? Is your partner happy too? Put this visit on your calendar like anything else, or you'll never do it!

Once you find a spiritual home, make every effort to stay committed to it. Try to set a good example for the kids and overlook any petty politics or cliquishness. Allow a steady practice of good deeds, right speaking, and appropriate involvement to help you find the people you want to hang out with. Go for depth instead of dabbling, going with the program instead of religion a la carte, and focusing on the big picture instead of shopping at the divine deli. Many a Cafeteria Catholic and Judgmental Jew, picking what to believe and rejecting the rest, has done some studying and been surprised by the pure spirituality and contemporary relevance behind beliefs they thought were old school. Popular adult Bat and Bar Mitzvah classes have educated a generation of boomers who were passed over as children for some reason, and these newly energetic Jews have become the superglue of synagogues. Check the leadership of the church service organization, and you'll usually find a Midlife Mama newly recommitted to keeping the faith.

Is there a women's study group? Go ahead and attend it as a prospective congregant, because this can be the source of amazing friendships and spiritual growth for you. If you don't actually want to join any congregation, sometimes you can still be a part of the women's group. As children move on, your options multiply.

I typed " women's bible study groups" into a search engine and hundreds of listings came up. An Adventist site about starting a new group had great ideas you could use for any denomination.

In my study group of Jewish women, the biggest problem is...well, studying. We make the wandering conversations on The *View* look scripted. We've been together so long that we can schmooz for hours about everything from world news to personal topics. Our wisest of Wise Women, Rona, will get us back on track by starting to read aloud, or I'll try a little positive promotion by quoting something in our text that's funny. The point of it all is that we are a little community of women of various ages who want to grow, and what could be better that that? Staying together is a priority, and we are flexible enough to schedule times and locations to accomplish that.

It's time to start thinking about the really big questions!

Is there a God? Does God answer prayer? Why are we here, what is my purpose? Why is there illness, suffering, and evil in the world? Why do bad things happen to good people? Why do people die? What happens after death, is there an afterlife? What is the afterlife like? What do I need to do to go to "the good place"?

Often, the only time we think about these questions is when a child asks them, or when someone close to us dies. Even if you know the position your religion takes on these questions, have you thought about how *you* feel about them? How sad, that we spend a lifetime making grocery lists and travel arrangements, but never ask or try to answer these questions. "It's just too big, I can't even go there!" you say, but imagine how you'd feel if you could safely read and talk about these things with friends, in pleasant surroundings. Imagine if you could reconnect with the bold little girl in your past who asked these questions without hesitation and expected an answer.

Rabbi Harold Kushner tracks the purpose of religion through our life stages in his book, *How Good Do We Have To Be?*

"When we are young, we turn to religion to help us find our way in the world, to make us prosperous, to make our dreams come true. When we reach middle age, we turn to religion to give us peace of mind and peace of soul. But when we grow old, we turn to religion to help us defeat death, our own and that of the people we love. We pray that the biopsy result will be favorable, that the surgery will succeed, that the illness will pass. And when we reluctantly conclude that God cannot keep us alive indefinitely no matter how good or pious we are, we ask Him to teach us to conquer death in another way, by giving us the blessing of memory...Only human beings can defeat death by summoning up the memory of someone they loved and lost, and feeling that person close to them as they do so."

The Checklist

❏ I. If you're thinking about becoming a minister or a rabbi, become a very active layperson in the congregation first. Work on yourself and get your own house in order before you run off to the seminary or yeshiva. See the organization from the inside out before you invest in your master's in theology. Read *The Year Mom Got Religion*, by Lee Meyerhoff Hendler, for a intimate preview of the joys and challenges of a midlife spiritual awakening.

❏ 2. Looking to work your way through the Bible? Going with a guide is more fun and efficient, smoothing you through the begats and priestly rulings. Christians look to the *Zondervan NIV Study Bible, Tyndale's Life Application Study Bible*, or Weaver's *Having a Mary Heart in a Martha*

World. Jews can learn the *Ancient Secrets*, by Rabbi Levi Meier, and Catholics will enjoy *The Catholic Youth Bible.*

❏ **3.** Great graduation gifts or interfaith bible study choices would be Kushner's *The Lord is My Shepherd* and *Complete Idiot's Guide to the Bible.* A delightful result of Christian theologian Harvey Cox's marriage to a Jewish woman is the book *Common Prayers*, an amazing resource in this age of interfaith marriage. Bring together Judaism, Islam, and Christianity in Feiler's *Abraham: A Journey to the Heart of Three Faiths.*

❏ **4.** Experience the perks of prayer starting today. Use your childhood prayer book to get started and then improvise from there. Have a nondenominational blessing in your Palm or planner at all times, so that no meal, meeting, or project need go unblessed. Always ask first, "Is it OK if I share a nondenominational blessing?"

❏ **5.** Start a walking group or exercise class at your house of worship and multi-task—you'll be getting healthier and associating with seekers at the same time.

The Checkup from the Neck Up

❏ I am consistent in my words, my thoughts, and my actions in my spiritual quest. Though I'm not perfect, I can be trusted to put one foot in front of the other and continue to grow at all times.

❏ I focus on joyful faith in my daily life, and as I go, I grow.

❏ I take full responsibility for my thoughts and choose to think only those thoughts which increase my faith and spiritual practice.

❏ I'm open to the spiritual strength that comes to me from new sources and I live each day with my mind searching for new paths to goodness and service.

33.

"To Pray is to Work, to Work is to Pray"

Believing that prayer heals the mind and the body is easy if we acknowledge that all acts of caring are prayers.

This "work is prayer" motto of the Benedictine order of monks reflects the attitude that prayer is actually part of the activities of daily life. When I remember my mother working in the kitchen for days at a time before a holiday, it's easy to believe that **all acts of caring are prayers**. The table set with the family's best dishes represents praise offered for the health and togetherness of the family, while the 3 a.m. vigil with a sick child is certainly a prayer for recovery. The sweet note to your lover, the compliment to a coworker, the meal sent to a sick neighbor can be seen as prayers of unity and recognition. In the book *Healing Beyond the Body*, Dr. Larry Dossey writes:

"Prayerfulness is more a matter of *being* than *doing*. I discovered that this makes sense to a lot of physicians. An eminent surgeon wrote me that after his medical and surgical training, he abandoned prayer and never formally prayed for his patients. Yet after thinking about the concept of prayerfulness, he realizes that he prays continually for his patients through his feelings of empathy, caring, and compassion for them – that, in fact, surgery for him is a continual exercise in prayer."

Dossey, a visionary physician and surgeon, makes a convincing argument for the idea that our power to heal and be healed extends beyond our bodies. He presents studies and anecdotes confirming that prayer, laughter, and love can all be powerful agents of healing. Dossey is the "cool guy" of the mind-body world, asking the questions you'd ask if you knew enough to wonder about it. He wonders, for example—what did the famous psychics, intuitives, and swamis die of? Why didn't they foresee their illness and heal themselves? This is in the same league as "Why don't we see the headline, 'Psychic Wins Lottery' very often?" but Dossey draws insightful conclusions even from this whimsical musing.

Prayer is to mind-body healing what walking is to exercise —anyone can do it and you don't need equipment. We don't even know if you have to believe in prayer for it to work, but most practitioners suggest that you fake it 'till you make it. If you don't know how to pray, find a book that appeals to you or, better yet, hang out with a prayerful person. As part of your daily walk, prayer synchs with breathing and the beauty of nature to send your good thoughts out into the cosmos. While driving or doing routine chores, turn your thoughts to beautiful and spiritual things, listen to a guided imagery or self talk CD, or lighten the day with your favorite spiritual music. Your thoughts and your actions are *both* prayers, kicking each other up a notch. Check out the Breathing Space gallery with soothing photos on Oprah.com, or the guided exercises on meditationcenter.com.

While driving with your family on a beautiful day, ask each person to describe what they think heaven is like—will loved ones separated by death be there? Will it be like a beachfront suite in Bali or a penthouse in Beverly Hills? Will we each have the fit, slim body we always wanted? Do pets go there? Can we eat whatever we want, when we want it, like on Star Trek? The fun and laughter of a conversation like this is a group prayer of the highest order, turning all thoughts to the rewards of right living. Like Dorothy's ability to go home in *The Wizard of Oz*, the power to heal and be healed has been within you all the time. Feel yourself lifted up, knowing that what you dwell on is what you become. Envision in joyful detail what health for you and your family looks like and what you will do with it.

Hand washing, aspirin, and penicillin were all proven effective as therapies before we understood exactly how they worked, just as what Dossey calls "intercessory prayer— communicating with the Absolute on behalf of sick people"—is now being tested in double-blind studies. Since 1988, several well-designed studies have shown that patients assigned to an intercessory (unknown) prayer group required less medication and had less severe symptoms. Can prayer be used like a drug? Can we point it like a gun at cancer cells and kill them? Or is prayer strictly a means of connecting with the sacred? Is it wrong to "use it" to attempt to control events?

"But why," you ask, "did we all pray for a loved one and she died? How could there be a 'higher good' involved when a child or young person dies?" To answer *those* questions, you must talk with people who share your traditions or background. Rough out your own story of why people leave this world, why there is suffering and pain, or finally become comfortable with *not* knowing why. Finding *your* answers to those tough questions is one of the tasks of midlife.

Just as we still can't really prove that the theory of gravity is a fact, Dr. Dossey writes that it may be a while before we can

empirically *prove* that prayer and other non-local methods can aid
traditional medicine in healing. Meanwhile, wouldn't it make sense
to add it to your arsenal of ways to care for yourself and others?

When you approach it in even the most superficial way, you
know that your thoughts affect your energy level and well
being. Contrast how tired you are on Monday morning when
the alarm wakes you for work with how you feel on Saturday
morning when you have an early tee-off time. Heart attack
rates are highest on Sunday evenings and Monday mornings.
When you take your Echinacea, does your cold go away
because you feel you've chased it, because of the supplements,
or some combination of both? Think about the rushing around
you do right before you're going on vacation; you feel excited
and happy, not tired. I see my friend Bobbi preparing for her
daughter's wedding, looking better than she has in the years
since her bout with breast cancer. When you got your sea legs
at a new job, remember how you jumped out of bed to greet
your new challenges (before you became familiar with the
recurring roadblocks)? Talking to your friend, positive reading,
and exercising make you feel less stressed, but think about the
Loser Zone activities you engage in to relieve your mind:
compulsive e-mail checking, net-surfing, shopping, and over
scheduling. All these everyday mind-games affect the body.

The wonderful physician/healers of our time—Drs. Herbert
Benson, Andrew Weil, Bernie Siegel, Deepak Chopra,
Christiane Northrup, Rachel Naomi Remen, and Larry Dossey,
among others—have taken observations about nontraditional
healing from their clinical practices and laid them out for us to
examine and learn from. Yes, they say, mind-body approaches
have eased suffering among men and women with almost any
medical condition. I think many of us gave lip service to
breathing techniques during our pregnancies, freaked out after

the first good contraction, and gave up on the whole category. But meditation techniques now have a long track record, and it's time to take a second look.

Girlfriends, this is not a new, untested, mystical idea! Since Dr. Herbert Benson introduced *The Relaxation Response* twenty-five years ago, millions of people have used this ridiculously simple technique to reduce everything from chest pains, blood pressure, and chemo nausea to headaches and anxiety. "The Science of Meditation" was recently a cover article in *TIME* magazine, saying that meditation is the "smart person's bubble bath" – is that mainstream enough for you? Dr. Benson shows the multiplying factor of combining the meditative response with "the faith factor," your personal beliefs, and the desire for health in his new book *Timeless Healing*. Though I'm no swami, I avoided drugs during two complicated deliveries using Lamaze breathing, and I also used the breathing techniques during painful procedures following a car accident. Major medical centers currently use guided imagery CD's by therapist Belleruth Naperstek for pre-surgery and recovery from cardiac procedures, chemotherapy, and trauma. You can use her CD's for weight loss and stress relief any old day; they're available on Amazon and other sites.

Women who are having hot flashes or premenstrual symptoms have a unique opportunity to test the mind-body connection. **That out-of-control feeling you get when you're having a hot flash or feeling depressed can be tamed by using relaxation techniques.** Using some version of the relaxation response, Alice Domar and other researchers at Harvard Medical School helped women tame their hot flashes by 50 % and PMS symptoms by 58%, lessening anxiety and depression in the process. Even women experiencing those notorious tamoxifen hot flashes had a 42% reduction.

What's meditation and/or the relaxation response? Simply put, it's taking 20 minutes each day to breathe deeply using your belly, empty your mind of everyday thoughts, and focus on or say an uplifting phrase as you slowly breathe in and out. The phrase could be spiritual—saying "Hail Mary" for Catholics, "Shalom" for Jews, or "His Grace" for Christians—or it could be a secular phrase like "we will/get there," "love," or "peace." You could combine meditation and affirmation to make it to your pregnancy's due date—"We will make it/ to October." If you find it impossible to quiet your thoughts, you might try the RESPeRATE biofeedback device detailed in Chapter 25. I find even RESPeRATE works better if you use a phrase to focus on.

> **"There are many things we can control that make us less vulnerable to illness. None of them comes in a pill."**
> Dr. Rachel Naomi Remen

When an elderly relative has multiple serious health challenges and a very limited lifestyle, do you ever wonder why they hang on to life so tenaciously? Do you think to yourself, "Would I want to live, if it was me?" Is it proof of the mind/body connection when a seriously ill person hangs on until a loved one arrives, or until they're told, "We'll be okay, you can go"? Dr. Remen's book *The Will to Live and Other Mysteries* explores this and many other questions about focusing on joy instead of illness, living fully and deeply, and acknowledging, "life is larger than science."

In all her books, this master storyteller, cancer specialist, and healer shows us what to look for in healing and in creating a huge, joyful life. She is an expert on how to recognize, feel entitled to, and receive blessings. "Blessing life may be more about learning to celebrate life than learning how to fix life…blessing life is about filling yourself up so that your blessings overflow onto others." I love the story this honored physician tells about hiding the ugly, dark pieces of a jigsaw puzzle when she was a little girl. She thought the family would have a more beautiful puzzle without them, but her mother shows her how the ugly pieces complete the puzzle, just as the dark places in our lives show us how valuable and important life is. After 30 years helping people heal and deal with cancer and 50 years of personally dealing with Crohn's disease, I'd say Dr. Remen qualifies as an expert on how to expand life instead of spending your life worrying about your health!

I've read customer reviews on Amazon that say they want to gag when they read this "New Age, mind/body healing, spiritual stuff." I used to feel the same way, back when I believed that you could exercise, take a pill, research the correct treatment on the Internet, and everything would be just perfect. But I've seen too many people wish they had other tools to use after they found the lump in their breast, the test came back positive, or they're in the Intensive Care Unit. Why wait? **As the saying goes, no one ever wishes on their deathbed that they'd spent more time at the office. Spend some time in meditation and calm prayer, appreciating the health God's given you.** Do you really need another research study to tell you about the health consequences of:

- dwelling on the past
- comparing yourself with others
- worrying constantly where the next buck will come from
- "dubbing in" what you imagine people think
- anticipating the worst at work, home, and play?

If it makes your stomach flutter just to read that list, imagine what a chronic habit of negative second-guessing does to your health. It can't be a good thing, and it certainly steals all the peace and joy out of the present! **The saying that you can't have fear and faith in the same body has consequences for your health.** Don't let the fear take up residence. Maybe the very act of learning to enjoy the present will deter the illnesses we fear; maybe it will just tick "regrets" off the list of things we'll have to deal with if the worst does happen.

When you start to take action and make decisions about your health, it's scary because you are also taking some responsibility for what may go wrong. That paralyzes some people. It may help to see yourself as becoming a partner to the medical professionals you work with, and, in the case of spiritual healing, as a partner to the Absolute you believe in.

The Checklist

❏ I. Massage therapy, acupuncture and pressure, guided imagery, yoga, and tai chi help people heal; hospitals often offer them and insurance may cover some procedures.

❏ 2. There are many effective variations on the meditation technique mentioned above: body scan relaxation (concentrating on body parts and letting go), progressive muscle relaxation (tightening and *then* letting go), mindfulness, guided imagery, and cognitive restructuring. These are detailed in *Healing Mind, Healthy Woman*, Alice Domar's excellent book that focuses specifically on using mind-body techniques in women's health.

❏ 3. If you like your mind-body learning with a dash of Eastern philosophy, you'll love Dr. Deepak Chopra's many books and videos, including *Perfect Health*. Caroline Myss's *Sacred Contracts and The Science of Medical*

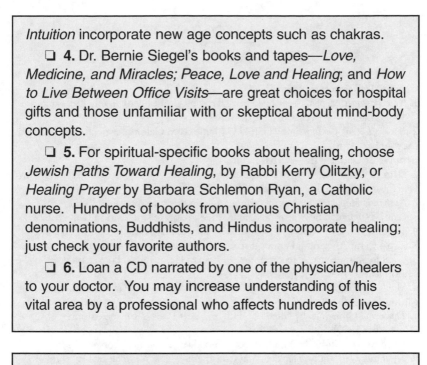

Intuition incorporate new age concepts such as chakras.

❏ **4.** Dr. Bernie Siegel's books and tapes—*Love, Medicine, and Miracles; Peace, Love and Healing*; and *How to Live Between Office Visits*—are great choices for hospital gifts and those unfamiliar with or skeptical about mind-body concepts.

❏ **5.** For spiritual-specific books about healing, choose *Jewish Paths Toward Healing*, by Rabbi Kerry Olitzky, or *Healing Prayer* by Barbara Schlemon Ryan, a Catholic nurse. Hundreds of books from various Christian denominations, Buddhists, and Hindus incorporate healing; just check your favorite authors.

❏ **6.** Loan a CD narrated by one of the physician/healers to your doctor. You may increase understanding of this vital area by a professional who affects hundreds of lives.

The Checkup from the Neck Up

❏ Every day, I become more full of peace, joy, and wisdom, no matter what the state of my health is.

❏ I am open to healing of all kinds, knowing that medical professionals may only have time to know their own areas.

❏ I am an active partner with everyone who can help me and my loved ones heal.

❏ I can fully focus on the present for a short time everyday, transcending reality by accepting it just as it is.

❏ I know that what we dwell on is what we become, so I often visualize the glowing health of those I love in my prayers and meditation.

❏ **I'm thrilled that I'm really starting to show the signs of aging—confidence, greater faith, wisdom, and strength!**

Credits

Chapter 1: Reinterpret your life story
1. *New Passages:Mapping Your Life Across Time* by Gail Sheehy, Joelle Delbourgo (Editor), Ballantine Books (Trd Pap); (June 1996)
2. *Love is Letting Go of Fear* by Gerald G., Jampolsky, Celestial Arts; Revised edition (September 1988)

Chapter 2: Garbage In—Garbage Out
1. *Learned Optimism, How to Change Your Mind and Your Life* by Martin Seligman, Free Press; Reissue edition (March 1998)
2. *Authentic Happiness* by Martin Seligman, Free Press; (September 2002)
3. *Learned Optimism* by Martin Seligman, Free Press; Reissue edition (March 1998)
4. *Magic Words: 101 Ways to Talk Your Way Through Life's Challenges,* by Howard Kaminsky and Alexandra Penney, Broadway Books, (November 2001)
5. *What to Say When You Talk to Yourself* by Shad Helmstetter, Pocket Books; Reissue edition (April 1990)
6. *Man's Search for Meaning* by Viktor Frankl, Pocket Books; Revised and Updated edition (December 1, 1997)
7. *Think and Grow Rich* by Napoleon Hill, Fawcett Books; Reissue edition (November 1990)
8. *Tuesdays with Morrie* by Mitch Albom, Broadway Books; (October 2002)
9. *The Power of Positive Thinking, You Can If You Think You Can* by Dr. Norman Vincent Peale, Fireside; (August 1987)
10. *Move Ahead with Possibility Thinking* by Robert H. Schuller, Jove Pubns; Reissue edition (December 1986)

Chapter 3—Lose Weight With Your Eyeballs
1. *Today I Am A Ma'am,* by Valerie Harper, Cliff Street Books, (April 2001)
2. *Don't Count the Candles: Just Keep the Fire Lit,* by Joan Rivers, Harper Torch, (May 2000)
3. *The Pocket Food and Exercise Diary,* by Allan Borushek, Family Health Pubs, (December 1996)
4. *The Better Life Institute,* BLIonline.com
5. *Atkins for Life,* by Robert C. Atkins, M.D., Random House, (June 2003)
6. *The Pritikin Weight Loss Breakthrough,* by Robert Pritikin, EP Dutton (January 1998)
7. *The South Beach Diet,* by Arthur Agatston, M.D., Bantam Books, (April 2003)
8. *Suzanne Somers' Fast and Easy,* by Suzanne Somers, Crown Pub Group, (December 2002)
9. *The RealAge Diet, Cooking the RealAge Way,* Drs. Michael F. Roizen & John La Puma, Harper Resource, (June 2003)
10. *Weight Watchers Make It In Minutes,* John Wiley & Sons, (August 2001)
11. *Nutrition Action Healthletter,* Center for Science in the Public Interest
12. *Slim to None,* Jennifer Hendricks, Comtemporary Books, January 2003

Chapter 4: Vitamin X
1. *Get With The Program,* by Bob Greene, Simon & Schuster; Spiral edition (January 2002)

2. *8 Minutes in the Morning*, by Jorge Cruise, HarperResource; (December 2002)
3. *Flip the Switch*, by Jim Karas, Harmony Books; 1st edition (December 2002)
Exercise videos available at collagevideo.com, Walmart, Costco and many other outlets

Chapter 5: Is Your Life Worth 30 Minutes a Day?
1. *Fit from Within*, by Victoria Moran, McGraw-Hill/Contemporary Books; (March, 2002)
2. *8 Minutes in the Morning*, by Jorge Cruise, Anthony Robbins (Foreword), HarperResource; (December, 2002)

Chapter 6: Devour and Conquer
1. *8 Weeks to Optimum Health*, by Andrew Weil M.D., Knopf (March 1997)
2. *Food: Your Miracle Medicine*, by Jean Carper, Harper Collins (1993)
3. Health Magazine
4. *Estrogen: The Natural Way*, by Nina Shandler; Villard (May 1998)
5. *A Dietitians Cancer Story*, by Diana Dyer 8th ed., Swan Press (April 2002)
6. *Nutrition Action Healthletter*—Soy Burger Review
7. *Maximum Food Power for Women*, by Julia Van Tine and Debra L. Gordon, Rodale Inc. (2001)

Chapter 7: If You Ate Like a Monkey
1. *Women, Weight, and Hormones*, Elizabeth Lee Vliet, M.D., M. Evans & Co, (2001)
2. *Bottled Water Rating*—Consumer Reports Magazine

Chapter 8: That Was Very 9/10 of You!
1. *The Lord is My Shepherd*, by Harold Kushner, Knopf, (August 2003)
2. *How Good Do We Have To Be*, by Harold Kushner, Little Brown & Co. (September 1997)
3. *The Sweet Potato Queens Book of Love*, *The Sweet Potato Queens Big-Ass Cookbook and Financial Planner*, by Jill Connor Browne, Three Rivers Press, (January 2003)

Chapter 9: Raising Kids: An endless essay
1. *Dick Enberg's Humorous Quotes for all Occasions*, by Dick Enberg with Brian and Wendy Morgan, Andrews McNeel Publishing; (2000)
2. *The Essential 55*, by Ron Clark, Hyperion; (May 2003)
3. *Good Kids, Difficult Behavior* by Joyce E. Divinyi & Elizabeth Fallon (Editor), Wellness Connection; (January 1997)
4. *Parenting Teens With Love and Logic*, by Foster W. Cline, Jim Fay, Navpress; (July 1993)
5. *Letting Go: A Parent's Guide to Understanding the College Years*, by Karen Levin Coburn, Madge Lawrence Treeger, Perennial Press; Third edition (July 1997)

Chapter 10: Empty Nesters and Boomerang Kids
1. *Birdbaths and Paper Cranes*, by Sharon Randall, Sleeping Bear Press; (September 2001)
2. *10 Insider Secrets to Job Hunting Success!*, by Todd Bermont, 10 Step Corporation; (December 2001)
3. *The Saving Graces*, by Patricia Gaffney, HarperTorch; (May 2000)
4. *Bridal Bargains: Secrets to Throwing a Fantastic Wedding on a Realistic Budget*, Denise and Alan Fields, Windsor Peak Press; 6th ed. (December 2002)
5. *All Grown Up:Living Happily Ever After With Your Adult Children*, by Roberta Maisel, New Society Publishers; (November 2001)

Chapter 11: Last Chance Midlife Mommies
1. *Conquering Infertility*, by Alice Domar Ph.D., and Alice Lesch Kelly, Viking Press (September 2002)

2. *Dr. Richard Marr's Fertility Book*, by Richard Marrs M.D., Lisa Friedman Block, Kathy Kirtland Silverman, Dell (March 1998)

Chapter 12: Husbands and Wives

1. *Life Strategies: Doing What Works, Doing What Matters*, Phillip C. McGraw, Ph.D, Hyperion, (January 2000)
2. *Men are from Mars, Women are from Venus*, by John Gray, HarperCollins; (April 1993)
3. *The Five Love Languages*, by Gary Chapman, Northfield Pub; (October 1992)
4. *When All You've Ever Wanted Isn't Enough*, by Harold Kushner, Fireside; (January 2002)
5. *Living a Life That Matters*, by Harold S. Kushner, Anchor Books; (August 2002)
6. *Fly Fishing Through the Midlife Crisis*, by Howell Raines, Anchor; (November 1994)
7. *The Divorce Remedy*, by Michele Weiner Davis, Simon & Schuster; (September 2002)
8. *The Verbally Abusive Relationship*, by Patricia Evans, Adams Media Corporation; 2nd edition (March 1996)
9. *Controlling People*, by Patricia Evans, Adams Media Corporation; (January 2002)
10. *Relationship Rescue*, by Phillip C. McGraw, Hyperion; (September 2001)
11. *Divorce and Money: How to Make the Best Financial Decisions During Divorce*, by Violet Woodhouse, Nolo Press; 6th edition (October 2002)
12. *When Love Dies*, by Judy Bodmer, Word Publishing; (July 1999)
13. *Hit Below the Belt*, by Ralph Berberich, M.D., Celestial Arts (March 2001)
14. *You Can't Make Love If You're Dead*, by Leon Prochnik, Ari Press, (December 2000)

Chapter 13: Losing Your Virginity

1. *Sex Over 50*, by Joel D. Block, Ph.D., and Susan Crain Bakos, Prentice Hall Press, (April 1999)
2. *Tickle Your Fancy: A Woman's Guide to Sexual Self-Pleasure*, by Sadie Allison, Tickle Kitty Press, (March 2001)
3. *Sex for One*, by Betty Dodson, Crown Publishing Group, (May 1992)
4. *For Women Only: A Revolutionary Guide to Overcoming Sexual Dysfunction and Reclaiming Your Sex Life*, by Jennifer Berman M.D., Laura Berman, Ph.D., Henry Holt & Co., (January 2001)
5. *Five Minutes to Orgasm Every Time You Make Love*, by Claire D.Hutchins, JPS Publishing, 2nd Revised Edition, (July 2000)
6. *Mars and Venus in the Bedroom: A Guide to Lasting Romance and Passion*, by John Gray, Ph.D., Perennial, Reprint Edition, (February, 1997)
7. *A Round-Heeled Woman: My Late-Life Adventure in Sex and Romance*, by Jane Juska, Villard, (May 2003)

Chapter 14: Sexual Fitness

1. Amy Bloom, "Feel the Heat" in the July issue of *O the Oprah Magazine*
2. *Making Love the Way We Used To...Or Better: Secrets of Satisfying Midlife Sexuality*, by Alan Altman, M.D. and Laurie Ashner, Contemporary Books, (2001)
3. *The Change Before the Change*, by Laura G. Corio, M.D.and Linda G. Kahn, Doubleday (January 2002)
4. *Women, Weight, and Hormones*, by Elizabeth Lee Vliet, M.D., M. Evans & Co. (October 2001)
5. *Sex Over 50*, by Joel Block, Ph.D., and Susan Crain Bakos, Prentice Hall Press, (April 1999)
6. *Sex, Sex, and More Sex*, by Sue Johansen, Regan Books (October 2003)

7. *How to Be a Great Lover: Girlfriend-to-Girlfriend Totally Explicit Techniques That Will Blow His Mind*, by Lou Paget, Broadway Books, January 1999

8. *Seductions: Tales of Erotic Persuasion*, by Lonnie Barbach, Ph.D., New American Library, (January 2000)

9. *52 Saturday Nights: Heat Up Your Sex Life Even More with a Year of Creative Lovemaking*, by Joan Elizabeth Lloyd, Warner Books (2000)

Chapter 15: What Goes Around Comes Around

1. *Phyllis Diller* quoted in Reader's Digest Magazine

2. *Elder Rage, or Take My Father...Please!*, by Jacqueline Marcel, Impressive Press, 2nd ed. (April 2003)

3. *Strong Women Stay Young; Strong Women, Strong Bones*, by Miriam Nelson, Perigee Press, July 2001

4. *"Wicked Stepmother"* from More Magazine

5. *Streetwise Retirement Planning: Savvy Strategies and Practical Advice for a Secure Financial Future*, by Lita Epstein, Adams Media Corporation (January 2003)

6. *Merck Manual*, by Mark Beers, Simon & Schuster, 2nd ed. (April 2003)

7. *The Complete Eldercare Planner*, by Joy Loverde, Times Books, 2nd ed. (April 2000)

Chapter 16: Friends Help You Love Your Life

1. *The Friendship Factor: How to Get Close to the People You Care For*, by Alan Loy McGinnis, Augsburg Fortress Publications, (May 1979)

2. *I Know Just What You Mean: The Power of Friendship in Women's Lives*, by Ellen Goodman and Patricia O'Brien, Fireside, (May 2001)

3. *The Reader's Choice: 200 Book Club Favorites*, by Victoria Golden McMains, Quill, (July 2000)

4. *The Reading Group Handbook: Everything You Need to Know to Start Your Own Book Club*, by Rachel W. Jacobsohn, Hyperion Revised Edition, (April 1998)

5. *The Lovely Bones*, by Alice Sebold, Little Brown & Co., 1st Edition (June 2002)

6. *The Red Tent*, by Anita Diamant, Picador USA, October 1998

Chapter 17: Soaring Solo

1. *Flying Solo: Single Women at Midlife*, by Carol Anderson, Susan Stewart and Sonia Dimidjian, WW. Norton & Co., Reprint Edition, (October 1995)

2. *The Rules for Online Dating: Capturing the Heart of Mr. Right in Cyberspace*, by Ellen Fein, Pocket Books (July 2002)

3. *Cast Your Net: A Step-by-Step Guide to Finding Your Soulmate on the Internet*, by Eric F. Fagan, Harvard Common Press (June 2001)

Chapter 18: Anything Worth Doing

1. *It's Only Too Late If You Don't Start Now*, by Barbara Sher, Delacorte Press; (April 13, 1999)

2. *What Color Is Your Parachute?*, by Richard Nelson Bolles, Ten Speed Press; (September 2002)

3. *Do What You Are*, by Paul D. Tieger, Barbara Barron-Tieger, Little Brown & Company; 3rd edition (April 2001)

4. *The Pathfinder: How to Choose or Change Your Career for a Lifetime of Satisfaction and Success*, by Nicholas Lore, Fireside; (January 1998)

5. *The Artist's Way*, by Julia Cameron, J. P. Tarcher; 10th edition (February 28, 2002)

6. *Women for Hire*, by Tory Johnson, Robin Freedman Spizman, Lindsay Pollack; Perigee; 1st edition (September 2002)

7. *The Complete Idiots Guide to the Perfect Resume,* by Susan Ireland, Alpha Books (Feb 2003)
8. *Use What You've Got & Other Business Lessons I Learned From My Mom,* by Barbara Corcoran with Bruce Littlefield, Portfolio, (February 2003)
9. *The Complete Guide to Second Homes for Vacations, Retirement, and Investment,* by Gary W. Eldred, John Wiley & Sons;(November 1999)

Chapter 19: It's My Perimenopause
1. *Screaming to be Heard,* by Elizabeth Lee Vliet M.D., M Evans & Co; 2nd edition (2001)
2. *Endometriosis: A Key to Healing Through Nutrition,* by Michael Vernon, Dian Shepperson Mills, Thorsons Pub; (September 2002)
3. *Healing Fibroids,* by Allan Warshowsky, Fireside; (August 2002)
4. *Your Guide to Hysterectomy, Ovary Removal, and Hormone Replacement: What All Women Need to Know,* by Elizabeth Plourde, New Voice Publications, (April 2001)
5. *The Woman's Guide to Hysterectomy:Expectations and Options,* by Adelaide Haas & Susan L. Puretz, Celestial Arts; Revised ed. (February 2002)
6. *Prevention* magazine, www.prevention.com, "Health information you can trust," Emmaus, PA
7. *What Your Doctor May Not Tell You About Premenopause,* by John R. Lee, M.D. with Jesse Hanley, M.D., Warner Books; (January 1999)
8. *Before the Change,* by Ann Louise Gittleman, Harper SanFrancisco; (February 1999)
9. *It's My Ovaries, Stupid!,* by Elizabeth Lee Vliet M.D., Scribner; (May 2003)

Chapter 20: Get It While You're Hot
1. *The Wisdom of Menopause,* by Christiane NorthrupM.D., Bantam Doubleday Dell Pub (Trd Pap); (January 2003)
2. "Den Mother to Zen Mother" & "free range person" from *Is It Hot in Here or Is It Me?,* by Gayle Sand, Perennial, Reprinted (May 1994)
3. *Women, Weight, and Hormones,* by Elizabeth Lee Vliet, M.D., M Evans & Co; (October 2001)
4. *Screaming to be Heard,* by Elizabeth Lee Vliet, M.D., M Evans & Co; 2nd edition (2001)

Chapter 21: Natural Hormones
1. *Screaming to be Heard: Hormone Connections Women Suspect and Doctors Still Ignore, Completely Revised and Expanded,* by Elizabeth Lee Vliet, M.D., M. Evans and Company, Inc.(2001)
2. *The Wisdom of Menopause: Creating Physical and Emotional Health and Healing*
3. *During the Change,* by Christiane Northrup, M.D., Bantam Books,(March 2001)
4. *The Change Before the Change: Everything You Need to Know to Stay Healthy in the Decade before Menopause,* by Laura G. Corio M.D. and Linda G. Kahn, Doubleday, (January 2002)
5. *What Your Doctor May Not Tell You about Menopause; What Your Doctor May Not Tell You about Premenopause,* by John R. Lee, M.D. and Jesse Hanley, M.D., Warner Books; (January 1999)
6. *The HRT Solution by Marla Ahlgrimm,* Avery Penguin Putnam; (August 1999) Also excellent, but published before recent HRT revelations:
7. *The Pause: Positive Approaches to Perimenopause and Menopause,* by Lonnie Garfield Barbach, Plume, Revised ed. (January 2000)

Chapter 22: Go With the Flow
1. *You Don't Have to Live With Cystitis,* by Larrian Gillespie, M.D., Avon; Revised and Updated edition (December 1996)

2. *Screaming To Be Heard*, by Elizabeth Lee Vliet M.D., M Evans & Co; 2nd edition (2001)
3. *The Wisdom of Menopause*, by Christiane Northrup, Bantam Doubleday Dell Pub (Trd Pap); (January 1, 2003)
4. *Women, Weight, and Hormones*, by Elizabeth Lee Vliet, M.D., M Evans & Co; (October 1, 2001)
5. *The Menopause Diet*, by Larrian Gillespie, M.D., Healthy Life Pubns; Revised edition (January 2003)

Chapter 23: Will Power and Your Financial Diet
1. Tucker quote from *Dick Enberg's Humorous Quotes for All Occasions*, by Dick Enberg with Brian and Wendy Morgan, Andrews McMeel Publishing (2000)
2. *The Two-Income Trap: Why Middle Class Mothers and Fathers Are Going Broke*, by Elizabeth Warren and Amelia Warren Tyagi, Basic Books (September 2003)
3. *The Millionaire Next Door: The Surprising Secrets of America's Wealthy*, by Thomas J. Stanley and William D. Danko, Pocket Books, Reprint Edition, (October 1998)
4. *Smart Women Finish Rich: 9 Steps to Achieving Financial Security and Funding Your Dreams*, by David Bach, Broadway Books, Revised Edition (January 2002)
5. *Managing To Be Wealthy*, by John E. Sestina, Dearborn Trade Publishing, (June 2000)
6. *Making the Most of Your Money*, by Jane Bryant Quinn, Simon & Schuster, Revised (November 1997)
7. *The Motley Fool Personal Finance Workbook: A Foolproof Guide to Organizing Your Cash and Building Wealth*, by David and Tom Gardner, Fireside, (December 2002)
8. *Personal Finance for Dummies*, by Eric Tyson, For Dummies, 4th Edition, (July 2003)
9. *The Road to Wealth: A Comprehensive Guide to Your Money*, by Suze Orman, Riverhead Books, (July 2001)
10. *Money Lessons for a Lifetime*, by Jim Jorgenson, Dearborn Trade Publishing (June 1997)

Chapter 24: Let Your Ripples Loose!
1. *The Cathedral Within: Transforming Your Life By Giving Something Back*, by Bill Shore, Random House Trade Paperbacks (November 2001)
2. *Get Outside: A Guide to Volunteer Opportunities and Working Vacations in America's Great Outdoors*, American Hiking Society, Falcon (March 2002)
3. *Alternatives to the Peace Corps*, by Jennifer S. Willsea & Megan Reule, Food First Books, 10th Edition (October 2003)
4. *Volunteer Vacations: Short-Term Adventures That Will Benefit You and Others*, by Bill McMillon, Doug Cutchins, and Anne Geissinger, Chicago Review Press, (February 2003)
5. *To Lead is to Serve: How to Attract Volunteers and Keep Them* by Shar McBee, Shar McBee Publisher, (February 1994)

Chapter 25: Newsflash about Heart Disease
1. *Women Are Not Small Men: Life-Saving Strategies for Preventing and Healing Heart Disease in Women*, by Nieca Goldberg, M.D., Ballantine Books (February 2003)
2. *The Better Life Institute Letter*, blionline.com
3. *Food: Your Miracle Medicine*, by Jean Carper, Harper Torch Reissue Edition, (June 1998)
4. *Maximum Food Power for Women: Harness the Natural Power of Food, Vitamins, and Herbs for Total Health and Well-Being*, by Julia Vantine & Debra L. Gordon, Rodale Press (January 2001)

Chapter 26: What's up Doc?
1. *Getting the Best From Your Doctor*, by Alan N. Schwartz, John Wiley & Sons; (December 1998)

2. *It's My Ovaries, Stupid!*, by Elizabeth Lee Vliet, M.D.,Scribner; (May 2003)
3. *Screaming to Be Heard*, by Elizabeth Lee Vliet, M.D., M. Evans & Co (2001)
4. *The Thyroid Solution*, Ridha Arem, M.D., Ballantine Publishing, (1999)

Chapter 27: Boning Up for Your Future
1. *Strong Women, Strong Bones: Everything You Need to Know to Prevent, Treat, and Beat Osteoporosis*, by Miriam Nelson, Ph.D., and Sarah Wernick, Perigee, Reissue Edition (July 2001)
2. *Osteoporosis: Prevention, Diagnosis & Management*, by Morris Nostelovitz, M.D., 4th Edition, Professional Communications (February 2003)

Chapter 28: Your Laugh Lines Prove You've Had More Fun
1. *Bobbi Brown's Beauty Evolution*, by Bobbi Brown, Harper Resource (October 2002)
2. *The Wrinkle Cure*, by Nicholas Perricone, M.D. Warner Books, (May 2001)
3. *The Wisdom of Menopause*, by Christiane Northrup, M.D., Doubleday (January 2003)
4. *The Youth Corridor*, by Gerald Imber, M.D., William Morrow, Reprinted Edition (May 1998) and online
5. *The Non-Surgical Facelift Book*, by Drs Michael Byun, William Truswell, & John Mendelsohn, Addicus Books, (May 2003)
6. *The Smart Woman's Guide to Plastic Surgery*, by Jean M. Loftus, M.D., Contemporary Books (January 1999)
7. *Two Girlfriends Get Real About Plastic Surgery*, by Susan J. Collini and Charlee Irene Ganny, Renaissance Books (March 2000)
8. *Secrets of a Beverly Hills Plastic Surgeon*, by Robert Kotler, M.D., Ernest Mitchell Publications (April 2003)

Chapter 29: Loss: Getting Beyond "Why Me?"
1. *I'd Rather Laugh*, by Linda Richman,Warner Books; (March 2002)
2. *The Widows Financial Survival Guide*, by Nancy Dunnan, Perigee, (June 2003)

Chapter 30: Start From the End and Look Back
1. *Tuesdays With Morrie*, by Mitch Albom & Stacy Creamer, Broadway Books, (October 2002)
2. *Your Money or Your Life*, by Joe Dominguez, Vicki Robin, Penguin USA (Paper); New edition (September 1999)
3. *Journaling to Save Your Life* by Michele Weldon, Hazelden Information Education; (September 2001)
4. *Conversations with God I, 11, &111*, by Neale Donald Walsch, Putnam Publishing Group; (January 1999)

Chapter 31: Have a Thick Skin and a Thin Heart
1. *Life Makeovers: 52 Practical and Inspiring Ways to Improve Your Life One Week at a Time*, by Cheryl Richardson, Broadway Books (December 2002)
2. *A Child Called "It:" One Child's Courage to Survive*, by Dave Pelzer, Health Communications, Reissue edition (October 1995)
3. *Letters to a Young Therapist*, by Mary Pipher, Ph.D. Basic Books (July 2003)

Chapter 32: Keeping the Faith
1. *A Woman's Worth* and *Everyday Grace: Having Hope, Finding Forgiveness, and Making Miracles*, by Marianne Williamson, Riverhead Books; (November 2002)
2. *Traveling Mercies*, by Anne Lamott, Anchor Books; (February 2000)
3. *How Good Do We Have To Be?*, by Harold S. Kushner, Little Brown & Co (Paper); (September 1997)

4. *The Year Mom Got Religion*, by Lee Meyerhoff Hendler, Jewish Lights Pub; (August 1999)

5. *Zondervan NIV Study Bible*, by Zondervan Bible Publishers, Zondervan; (October 2002)

6. *Life Application Study Bible*, by Tyndale House Publishers, Tyndale House Publishers; (June 1997)

7. *Having a Mary Heart in a Martha World: Finding Intimacy with God in the Busyness of Life*, by Joanna Weaver, Waterbrook Press; Revised paper edition with new bible study (April 2002)

8. *Ancient Secrets: Using the Stories of the Bible to Improve Our Everyday Lives*, by Rabbi Levi Meier, Jewish Lights Publishing; (September 1999)

9. *The Catholic Youth Bible, New Revised Standard Version; Catholic Edition*, by Brian Singer-Towns (Editor), St. Mary's Press; (February 2000)

10. *Common Prayers: Faith, Family, and a Christian's Journey Through the Jewish Year*, by Harvey Cox, Mariner Books; (November 2002)

11. *Complete Idiot's Guide to the Bible*, by James S. Bell, Stan Campbell, James S., Jr. Bell, Jody P. Schaeffer, Alpha Books; 2nd edition (July 2002)

12. *Abraham: A Journey to the Heart of Three Faiths*, by Bruce Feiler, William Morrow; 1st edition (September 2002)

Chapter 33: To Pray is to Work and to Work is to Pray

1. *Healing Beyond the Body* by Larry Dossey, M.D., Random House, (October 2001))

2. *The Relaxation Response*, by Herbert Benson, Miriam Z. Klipper, HarperTorch; Reissue edition (November 2000)

3. *Timeless Healing* by Herbert Benson, Marg Stark, Scribner; Reprint edition (April 1997)

4. *The Will to Live and Other Mysteries,*, by Rachel Naomi Remen, M.D. Sounds True; unabridged edition (April 2001)

5. *Healing Mind, Healthy Woman*, by Alice D. Domar, Ph.D, Henry Dreher, Delta; (September 1997)

6. *Perfect Health*, by Deepak Chopra, M.D., Three Rivers Press; Revised and Updated edition (February 2001)

7. *Sacred Contracts*, by Caroline Myss, Three Rivers Press; 1st edition (January 2003)

8. *The Science of Medical Intuition*, by Caroline Myss, Sounds True; Unabridged edition (November 2002)

9. *Love, Medicine, and Miracles*, by Bernie S. Siegel, Perennial Press; Reissue edition (September 1998)

10. *Peace, Love and Healing*, by Bernie S. Siegel, Perennial Press; Reprint edition (September 1998)

11. *How to Live Between Office Visits*, by Bernie S. Siegel, Perennial Press; Reprint edition (April 1994)

12. *Jewish Paths Toward Healing*, by Rabbi Kerry M. Olitzky, Jewish Lights Pub; (August 2000)

13. *Healing Prayer*, by Barbara Schlemon Ryan, Vine Books, (September 2001)

Index

AAA, 221
AARP, 2,102,220,221
A Child Called It, 290
A Woman's Worth, 294-295
Abraham: Journey to the Heart of Three Faiths, 302
Acupuncture, 310
Activella, 203
Actonel, 261
A Dietitian's Cancer Story, 64
Adoption,106-108
Adult acne, 268-269
Ahlgrimm, Marla, 206
Albom, Mitch, 19, 281
Aldactone, 187
Altman, Dr. Alan, 136
Alternatives to the Peace Corps, 235
Alzheimers, 51,147-148, 193,238,240,253,
American Heart Association, 241,244
Angioplasties, 238
Antibiotics, 71, 222
Antidepressants, 33,198-199, 243,269
Arginmax, 139
A Round-Heeled Woman, 135
Artistry, (Time Defiance 100, 267)
    (Bright Idea, AlphaHydroxy 267)
Artist's Way, 171
Aspirin, 240
Astroglide, 137,205
Atkins diet, 28-30
Atridox, 269
Avage, 267
Avlimil, 139
Bach, David, 220
Barbach, Lonnie, 151
Beano, 61
Before the Change, 189
Benson, Dr. Herbert, 193,307
Berman, Dr. Jennifer,126,214
Berman, Dr. Laura,126
Better Life Institute, 28,238
Bible, 293-302
Bioidentical Hormones, 202-220,268
Birdbaths and Paper Cranes, 95
Birth control pills, 195-196
Black cohosh, 74-75
Block, Joel D., 124,151
Bloating, 198

Bloom, Amy,134
Bobbi Brown, 263, 265
Bobbi Brown's Beauty Evolution, 263
Book groups,160
Botox,270
Braun Oral B, 269
Bridal Bargains, 104
BriteSmile, 270
Buffet, Warren, 236
Calcium, 59,68,182,256-262
Cameron, Julia, 171
Cancer, 209-209
Cardiovascular disease, 249-260
Career development, 179-189
Carper, Jean, 59-60
Cathedral Within, 233
Catholic Youth Bible, 302
Celexa, 256
Cialis,143
Change Before the Change, 139,146
Change Your Career, 135
Chapman, Gary, ll6
Checkup checklists, 248-257
Chelation, 244
Cholesterol, 238-246
Chopra, Deepak, 306,310
Clearlight, 269
Climara, 136, 202,204, 273
COBRA, 104
Colonoscopy, 261,265,270
Collage.video.com, 49
Conversations with God, 287
Common Prayers, 302
Complete Eldercare Planner, 151
Complete Idiot's Guide to Perfect Resume, 173
Condoms,168
Conner, Jill, 81
Conquering Fertility, 108
Consumer Reports, 42
Controlling People, 121
CoQ10, 73,76, 186
Corio, Dr. Laura, 139,217
Cosmoplast,cosmoderm,270
Cozaar, 244
Cranberry juice, 224
Crestor, 257
Credit cards, 227-230
CRP, 264

Cruise, Jorge, 30-31,38,49,55
Cymbalta, 198
Dannon Light 'n Fit, 61
Davis, Michelle Weiner, 119
Depression, 73, 84-86
Dating, 163-168
DEXA, 258-262
DHEA, 200
Diane 35, 195
Differin, 283
Disability insurance, 232
Divorce and Money, 122
Divorce Remedy, 119
Domar, Alice, 108,307
Dossey, Dr. Larry 303-306
Downey Side America, 107
Dr. Richard Marr's Fertility Book, 108
Echinacea, 72
Effexor, 192
Eight Minutes in the Morning, 29-30,36,46,54
Eight Weeks to Optimum Health, 57
Elder Rage, 147
Endometriosis, 185
Enova oil, 35,63
Erection,145,146,148,150
Essential 55, 88
Essure technique, 189
Estrace, 137,202,204, 211
Estradiol, 143, 144,191-208, 254, 260-262
Estradiol patch, 199,200,203,204
estragel, 214
Estratest, 139
Estring,137,204-205
Estring, 205,216-217
Estriol,137,204,211
Estrogen: the Natural Way, 63
Ephedra, 77
Essential 55, 92
Equity loan,229-230
Evans, Patricia, 121
Everyday Grace, 310
Exercise, 37-58,148,250
Faith, 310-327
Fake Bake, 266
Femring, 204
Fibroids, 184-185
Financial planners, 233
Financial web sites, 233
Fish oil, 64, 73,260
Fit from Within, 49
Five Love Languages, 116
Five Minutes to Orgasm Every Time You Make Love, 127
Flax, flaxseed oil, 31, 35,64-65,66,73,189

Flip the Switch, 30,46
Fly Fishing Through the Midlife Crisis, 114
Flying Solo,162
Food: Your Miracle Medicine, 57-58
FSH, 201
Forgiveness, 303-307
For Women Only, 126,214
Fosamax, 261
Frankl, Victor 19
Friendship Factor, 152
Frequent flyer miles, 247
Funeral, 293-294
Gaffney, Patricia, 102
Garlic, 76-77
Get Outside, 235
Getting the Best From Your Doctor, 262
Get With the Program, 31-32,37,49
Gillespie, Dr. Larrian 209-214
Gittleman, Ann Louise, 189
Gingko, 76
Glucosamine, 75
Goldberg, Nieca, 236
Good Kids, Difficult Behavior, 88
Greene, Bob, 30,35,36
Grey, John, 109, 127
Grief, 112, 292
Gynodial, 202
Hanley, Dr. Jesse,206
Harper, Valerie, 21
Having a Mary Heart in a Martha World, 301
Hawthorn, 260
Healing Beyond the Body, 303
Health insurance, 104, 108
Health Magazine, 19,58,257
Heart attack, 237
Helmstetter, Shad,17
Hit Below the Belt, 122
Hollywood Tan, 265
Homeopathy, 74
Hopewell Pharmacy, 268
Hormone replacement, 254, levels, 266, general 202-220, for heart, 241, for skin and hair, 268
Hot flashes, 71,72,183,188
How Good Do We Have To Be?, 80,301
How to Be A Great Lover, 144
HRT, 195-197,241
Humor, 84-85
Hypertension, high blood pressure, 239-247
Hysterectomy, 185-186
I'd Rather Laugh, 275
Interstitial cystitis, 210-215
It's My Ovaries, Stupid!,189
Imber, Dr.Gerald, 271

Incontinence, 209-214
Intrinsa, 139,218
Investments, 215-230
Is it Hot in Here, Or is it Me? 195
It's Only Too Late If You Don't Start Now, 169
Ivillage, 75
Jampolsky, Dr. Gerald, 7
Johanson, Sue,148, 151
Journaling, 285-286
Journaling to Save Your Life, 287
Juska, Jane, 128
Karas, Jim, 30, 46
Karper,Jean,58
Kashi, 62
Kegels, 137,223
Kidsave.com, 107
Kotler, Dr. Bob, 272
Kushner, Harold, 78, 80, 113, 301, 318
KY jelly, 137
Lamott, Anne, 295
Learned Optimism, 9
Lee, Dr. John R., 206
LegalZoom.com, 220
Letters to a Young Therapist, 290
Letting Go, 91-92
Levitra,143
Life Makeovers, 288
Life Strategies, 109
Lloyd, Joan Elizabeth, 151
Long term care insurance 221
Lord is My Shepherd, 78, 318
Loss, 275-280
Love is Letting Go of Fear, 7
Lyme disease, 257
Magic Words, 13
Making the Most of Your Money, 224
Making Love the Way We Used To, 135-136
Male menopause, 118
Mammogram, 256
Managing to be Wealthy, 223,229
Man's Search for Meaning, 19
Margerine, 63
Mars and Venus in the Bedroom, 127
Massage, 326
Masturbation, 133
McBee, Shar 235
McGinnis, Alan Loy,152
McGraw, Dr. Phil, 93, 109,122
Medical web sites, 263
Meditation, 38,307-311
Melanotan, 140
Men are from Mars, Women are from Venus, 109
Menopause, 191- 214
Men's Health, 19

Merck Manual, 151
Mevacor, 239
Midlife crisis, 113
Mifepristone, 184
Migraines, 77,80,186-187
Milk thistle, 76
Millionaire Next Door, 218
Mind-Body Healing, 319-327
Minkin, Dr. Mary Jane, 187
Moran, Victoria, 49
More Magazine, 19,149
Motley Fool Personal Finance, 224
Move Ahead with Possibility Thinking, 19
Movie selections, 159
Myss, Caroline, 311
Mystic Tan, 279
Nail fungus, 287
Naperstek, Belleruth, 307
National Adoption Information
    Clearing House, 107
Nature Made Cholestoff, 239
Nelson, Dr. Miriam, 148
Neocontrol, 211
*New Passages: Mapping Your Life
    Across Time,* 1
Niacin, 239
Nicotine replacement, 242-243
Non-ablative lasers, 267
Non-Surgical Facelift Book, 271
Northrup, Dr. Christiane, 139,191,196,268
NTx, 275
Nutrition Action Healthletter, 32,58
Nutrilite - green tea Cholesterol
    Health 239, CLA 77, CoQ10 70,
    Glucosamine 72, Naturally
    Together 140, Protein Bars 32,
    Digestive Enzyme Complex 59,
    (XX & Leading Edge 67), quality of
    69-70, (PMS Plus & Black
    Cohosh 71), (Milk Thistle &
    Siberian 73), Saw Palmetto 122
Olitzky, Rabbi Kerry, 311
Omega 3's, 61-62,72-73
Oprah.com, Oxygen, 7
Oral contraceptives, 183-184
Orgasm, 124-144
Ortho-Cyclen, 184
O the Oprah Magazine, 19, 134
Osteoporosis, 258-262
Ovcon 35, 184
Paget, Lou,144
Parenting Teens with Love & Logic, 90
Pathfinder: How to Choose Career, 171
Paxil, 84,187-188, 243

Pedometer, 46
Penney, Alexandra & Howard Kaminsky, 13
Perimenopause, 180-190
Perricone, Nicholas, 267
Personal Finance for Dummies, 224
Pharmacies, 205,207
Pilates, 37-38
Pravachol, 239
Prayer, 17,310-327
Premarin, Prempro, 194-195, 254,274
Premenstrual syndrome, 51, 73,191-204
Prevention, 19, 25,32,44,60,187
Pritikin diet, 28
Procheive gel, 150,202,204
Progest, 215
Progesterone,261,191-208
Prometrium, 202-204
Prozac, 84, 139,187-188,192,243
Psychologists & psychiatrists, 86-87
Psyllium, 259
Quicken Lawyer 2003, 219
Quixtar, XS-33, 76,
    (Quickflex &Magnabloc, 46),
    Ocean Essentials 70, e-Spring filter 75
Randall, Sharon, 95
Reader's Digest, 19
Real Age Diet, 31
Real Simple, 284
Relaxation Response, 182,307
Remen, Dr. Rachel Naomi, 306, 308-309
Replens, 137
Resperate, 241,308
Retinol, 281
Revival Soy, 32,140
Richardson, Cheryl, 288
Richman, Linda, 275
Ritter, John, 55
Road to Wealth, 224
Rosacea,269
Sand, Gayle, 195
Sansone, Leslie, 45,148
Sasaki, Dr. Gordon, 287
Saving Graces, 102
Sawyer,Diane,30,264
Schiff's Prostate Health, 128
Screaming to be Heard,
    136,183,201,206,220,225
Seasonale, 184
*Secrets of a Beverly Hills Cosmetic
    Surgeon*, 272
Seligman, Dr. Martin, 9-12
Sestina, John, 219,223,226,229
Sex and the City, 166
Sex, Sex, and More Sex, 144

Sex Over 50, 124,151
Shabbat, 284
Shandler, Nina, 63
Sheehy, Gail, 1
Sher, Barbara, 169
Shock Absorber bra, 49
Shore, Bill 233
Siegel, Dr. Bernie, 311
Silken Secret,144
Simplify, 297-298
Sleep, 78-79
SleepRight Mouth Guard, 273
Slim to None, 35
Smart Woman's Guide to Plastic Surgery, 285
Smart Women Finish Rich, 242-243
Smoking, 242-243
Solaray Red Yeast Rice, 252
Somersizing, 28-29,33
South Beach Diet, 28-29
Soy, 63-65,200
Soy burgers, 67
Splenda, 33
Statin drugs, 238-239
St. John's Wort, 76,188
Streetwise Retirement Planning, 151
Strokes, 237
Strong Women, Strong Bones, 148
Sunday Night Sex Show, 144
Supplements, 69-80
Suze Ormond's Protection Portfolio, 232
Sweet Potato Queens Book of Love, 81
Teens, 92-95
Term life insurance, 232,233
The Firm, 49
Thyroid, 252
Today I Am A Ma'am, 21
To Lead is to Serve, 235
Travel web sites, 241
Tri-Luma, 268
Ten Insider Secrets to Job Hunting, 104
Testosterone, 137,218
ThermaCool, 269,270
Thiazide diuretics, 254
Think and Grow Rich, 19
Thyroid, 265
Tickle Your Fancy, 126
Today Sponge, 189
Transdermal patch, 211,212,216
Traveling Mercies, 295
Triage Cardiac System, 269
Tubal ligation, 200,201
Tuesdays with Morrie, 19, 281
*Two Girlfriends Get Real About Plastic
    Surgery*, 271

Ultrawhite, 273
Urinary tract, 209-214
USA Today, 19
US News and World Report, 178
Vagifem, 137,204-205,211
Vaginal atrophy, 136,204-205
Valerian, 71
Verbally Abusive Relationship, 121
Viactiv, 273
Viagra, 142-143
Vitamin C creams, 267
Vitamin K, 76,268
Vitamin supplements, for heart
    health 246-247, General, 69-80
Vitex, 74
Vivelle, 136, 202,203,261
Vliet, Dr. Elizabeth Lee, 66,139,183,
    189,193194,197,200,201,203,208,214
Volunteer, 244-247
Volunteer Vacations, 235
Walking, 45-47
Water, 77
Websites, health 250,finance 221
Weight Control,20-34
Weight Watchers, 31
Weil, Andrew, 57
Wellbutrin, 84,188,243
What to Say When You Talk to Yourself, 17

When Love Dies, 128
Williamson, Marianne, 294
Wills, 230-232
Winfrey,Oprah, 202
Wisdom of Menopause, 135,191,196,214
Wodehouse, Violet P., 128
Woman's Day, 19
Women Are Not Small Men, 236
Women, Weight, and Hormones,
    66,146, 193,200,214
Women for Hire, 172
Worst Pills, Best Pill, 257
Wrinkle Cure, 267
Wrinkle fillers, 284
Women are not Small Men, 249
Womens Health Initiative,
    194-198,207,237
Yasmin, 184, 283
Year Mom Got Religion, 317
Yoga, 39-40
You Can't Make Love If You're Dead, 122
You Don't Have to Live With Cystitis, 211-214
Youth Corridor, 271
Zestra, 140
Zetia, 239
Zocor, 238-239
Zoloft, 84,85,198
Zoom, 270

Quick Order Form

Online orders: Visit our store to order books and other
Midlife Mamas merchandise: www.midlifemamas.com
Fax orders: Using this form for credit card orders. 877-609-3718

Postal orders: Fast Forward Publications
P.O. Box 573
Long Valley, N.J. 07853
(Use this form and send along with
check or credit card information)

Name: _____

Address _____

City _____   State ____   Zip _____

Telephone: _____

Email address:_____

_____Quantity   _____Total
@ \$14.95 U.S. funds each
\$29.95 Can.   _____Shipping & handling

          _____Tax (NJ residents only 6%)

Shipping and Handling: \$4.00 for 1 - 4 books
          \$6.00 for 5 - 10 books
Quantity discounts available over 10 books—contact us

Payment: ❑ check or money order
       ❑ Visa   ❑ Mastercard   ❑ AMEX   ❑ Discover

Card Number: _____

Name on Card: _____   Exp. date: _____

Also available: Keynote speaking
          Midlife Mamas seminars and workshops

Contact us at speaking@midlifemamas.com or the address above.